Generational Intelligence

The question of communication and understanding between different generations is emerging as a key issue for the twenty-first century. The advent of ageing populations may lead to increased conflict or solidarity in society, and provokes a profound ambivalence both in the public and in the private sphere. In a new approach, Biggs and Lowenstein offer a critical examination of Generational Intelligence as one way of addressing these issues. How easy is it to put yourself in the shoes of someone of a different age group? What are the personal, interpersonal and social factors that affect our perceptions of the 'age other'? What are the key issues facing families, workplaces and communities in an ageing society? This book sets out a way of thinking about interpersonal relations based on age, and the question of communication between people of different ages and generations. The book challenges existing orthodoxies for relations between adults of different ages and draws out steps that can be taken to increase understanding between generational groups. The authors outline a series of steps that can be taken to enhance Generational Intelligence, examine existing theories and social issues, and suggest new directions for sustainable relations between generational groups.

Simon Biggs is Professor of Gerontology and Social Policy at the School of Social and Political Sciences, University of Melbourne, Australia, and Visiting Professor at the Institute of Gerontology, King's College London, UK.

Ariela Lowenstein is Professor and Head of the Center for Research and Study of Ageing at the Faculty of Welfare and Health Studies, University of Haifa, Israel.

Generational Intelligence

A Critical Approach to Age Relations

Simon Biggs and Ariela Lowenstein

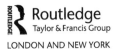

LONDON AND NEW YORK

First published 2011
by Routledge
2 Park Square, Milton Park, Abingdon, Oxon, OX14 4RN

Simultaneously published in the USA and Canada
by Routledge
711 Third Avenue, New York, NY 10017

Routledge is an imprint of the Taylor & Francis Group, an informa business

© 2011 Simon Biggs and Ariela Lowenstein

British Library Cataloguing in Publication Data
A catalogue record for this book is available from the British Library

Library of Congress Cataloging in Publication Data
Biggs, Simon J.
  Generational intelligence : age, identity, and the future of gerontology /
  Simon Biggs and Ariela Lowenstein.
    p. ; cm.
  Includes bibliographical references and index.
  1. Gerontology. 2. Identity (Psychology) 3. Generations.
  I. Lowenstein, Ariela. II. Title.
  [DNLM: 1. Aged—psychology. 2. Intergenerational Relations.
  3. Emotional Intelligence. 4. Geriatrics. 5. Negotiating. WT 145]
  HQ1061.B527 2011
  305.26—dc22
                                  2010040386

ISBN: 978–0–415–54654–6 (hbk)
ISBN: 978–0–415–54655–3 (pbk)
ISBN: 978–0–203–82791–8 (ebk)

Typeset in Times New Roman by Swales & Willis Ltd, Exeter, Devon

Contents

Preface

This book was born from a long-standing professional collaboration and exchange of ideas between the two authors on various issues in social gerontology. Both of us come from different social science disciplines and trained in different methods – Biggs in social psychology and qualitative work and Lowenstein in sociology and quantitative methods. Both have had an enduring interest in social issues and problems as they affect adult life. Both have also worked in social work, one with an emphasis on psychodynamic and the other on family approaches. Thus, we arrive at this endeavour from different disciplinary orientations and intellectual perspectives, debating a variety of concepts and viewpoints that have been commonly encountered. Each of us has his/her own writing style which has added creativity to the task, and is also reflected in the book. We had many meetings throughout the three years of writing, which were essential for the negotiation of ideas and the engaging process of trying to develop a new approach to intergenerational relations. The face-to-face meetings were important in order for us to share perspectives, provoke each other, generate ideas and iron out differences. We discovered that collaboration is more challenging than is usually thought and that it is a multidimensional and multi-method process which itself takes time to take shape.

Our collaboration has culminated in the theoretical thinking evidenced in the current book. We have built on, but also reconstructed existing debates and in so doing hope to have created a space in which a new concept has taken shape, namely that of Generational Intelligence. The book is, then, about the process of research and thinking about intergenerational relations, focusing on studies already undertaken in this area, the construction of existing work and limits of knowledge. It is also about new conceptual thinking to advance that knowledge. As part of this we explore the meaning of generation, the connection between ageing and generation, relations between generational groups; distinctions and interactions between cohort, family, and life position, agency and social structure. We then discuss a number of key topics through the lens of that novel concept, perhaps in a generationally intelligent manner.

The book should be useful to scholars, professionals and students working in the area of adult ageing and intergenerational relations.

Acknowledgements

Both authors would like to thank the many people, colleagues and students, who have listened to, commented on and contributed to the various ideas and presentations that have been incorporated in the book.

We also want to acknowledge the smooth and substantively helpful working relationship we have experienced with Routledge.

We would like to extend special thanks to Mrs Sigal Naim, a graduate with honors of the MA Department of Gerontology and Coordinator of the Center for Research and Study of Aging at the University of Haifa, Israel, who helped with the final editing, referencing and collation of the manuscript.

In particular, Simon Biggs would like to thank Irja Haapala, Guy Biggs and Eve Allen for their continued inspiration and support. He would also like to thank Taina Rantanen and staff at the University of Jyvaskyla, where he found time and space to write, and colleagues at the Institute of Gerontology, King's College London, for their forbearance while he was on sabbatical.

Ariela Lowenstein wants to thank her husband Ami for his ongoing enthusiasm about the book, support and encouragement all through the years of writing, and to thank her children Noam, Ruth and Tal and their spouses for being there for her.

Introduction

Rarely have societies witnessed a 'silent revolution' of such significance as the global phenomenon of population ageing (Kinsella, 2000; WHO, 2007), which impacts generational relationships and changes the landscape of individuals, families and societies. During the last decades, there has been unprecedented growth in the number and proportion of older persons in most countries around the world, a trend which is expected to continue. This reflects a globalization of issues associated with adult ageing, even though the pace is more gradual in some countries and more rapid in others (Bengtson *et al.*, 2003). Worldwide, the proportion of people aged 60 years and over is increasing faster than any other age group. In 2025, there will be a total of about 1.2 billion people 60 years and older (WHO, 2007). Thus, population ageing is a major factor impacting intergenerational relations and changes within these relationships. This shift in the demographic map needs to be located in broader social developments and in the way people think about generations in their personal lives.

Intergenerational relations cover different levels of social units such that micro-level interpersonal relations and macro-level structures and policies do not stand alone but interact (Walker, 1996). Such interaction, which includes the relationship between public and private spheres and between social and personal experience, offers a useful arena for analysing relations within and between generations. As Connidis and McMullin (2002a) state: 'Individuals as actors exercise agency as they negotiate relationships within the constraints of social structure' (p. 558). In other words, people have a degree of choice and autonomy, but this always has to be negotiated within existing prefiguring arrangements which are not always of their own choosing.

In this book, our main goal has been to develop a new conceptual-theoretical framework for understanding intergenerational relations in their broadest perspective.

We believe that 'theorizing is a process of developing ideas that allow us to understand and explain our data'(Bengtson *et al.*, 2005: 4). Theory provides

> Fundamental orienting perspectives for how questions are asked and solutions formulated . . . It may also provide conceptual tools to interpret complex events and critically evaluate the current state of affairs. . . . At the extreme

end of theory building, the ideas and explanations are infused with novelty and open new directions.

(Biggs *et al.*, 2003: 2, 7)

In our case, knowledge about the complex and multidimensional topic of intergenerational relations would expand horizons that are being shaped by and attempting to anticipate changing demographics and cultural demands on social systems, families and individual life courses. We are living in times when a paradigm shift is emerging in relations between generations which need new tools to explain and understand it. One example of such change comes from the OASIS[1] study, in which both authors were involved, one as lead researcher and the other as an outside adviser. The findings indicated that norms of support between generations have a sufficiently open character to allow an accommodation to new social realities and new forms of relationship. As gender equality and increased female participation in work-life impact family intergenerational relationships, families are becoming less duty driven and more open to negotiation. Affection and attachment emerged as more important for family cohesion and intergenerational ties, lending family relationships a more personal and a less structural flavour (Lowenstein and Daatland, 2006). Here, we attempt an outline of some of the key issues and contradictions in this field and achieve a new path for thinking about an increasingly important development and some of the social issues that emerge from it.

The first area that we would like to address, in this introductory chapter, concerns the concept of 'generation' where 'the conceptual language surrounding it is itself confusing' (Phillipson, 2010: 14). Generation has been referred to as a 'packed social concept' (McDaniel, 2008), including a variety of social, familial and personal associations, that influence personal identity. Bengtson and Putney (2006) argue that: 'The problem of generations and ageing represents one of the most enduring puzzles about social organization and behavior' (p. 20).

Hagestad and Uhlenberg (2007) discuss three different phenomena assigned to this term: first, age groups or individuals as given life stages; second, historical generations defined as birth cohorts with specific attributes; and third, family generations – locations in a system of ranked descent. These authors outline that:

In focusing on these three, one is examining people who not only are anchored differently in dimensions of time, primarily biographical time/chronological age and historical time but also the rhythm of family time. . . . A host of challenging yet neglected issues lies in the intersection of these three phenomena.

(Hagestad and Uhlenberg, 2007: 239–40)

Later in the book we look at the phenomenology of generation, and how, rather than starting out from thinking in terms of cohorts, families and individual life positions, people experience generation 'all in one go'. This implies both a holistic experience and one that is often tacit rather than consciously thought through.

Generation is, then, an amalgam of influences that may not be directly accessible to experience. It nevertheless underpins much of everyday attitudes and behaviour. We are generational beings in a variety of ways. We are by virtue of being temporal creatures, ones that develop over time and thus subject to processes of increasing maturity and the accumulation of experience. Our internal world therefore, comes to include associations, images and identifiable figures that are generationally inflected. These processes both distinguish individuals from each other and form the basis for shared generational experiences.

In addition, most people grow up in families that consist of different generations. Even for those who do not, the surrounding culture, its institutions and opportunities for self- expression are generationally organized. The influences of family on intergenerational relationships are picked up again later in the book. Here, concern lies with its effect on personal identity as one's earliest memories and attempts to define who one is, are formed in relation to familial others. Such influences embed themselves within us before we have the verbal tools to articulate what is happening, separate them out and achieve a critical distance from them. Sometimes, these relations are so pervasive that the ability to distinguish oneself from others can be lost, perspectives cease to be specific and dominant ways of perceiving eclipse those that are less powerful.

Finally, individuals may begin to realize that as they are striving to define themselves and their place in society, they are part of a stream of others who, having been born at the same time, in the same historical, cultural or social circumstances, are travelling the same paths. These pathways, may become culturally labeled, as the 'war generation', 'baby-boomers' or the 'millennium children' and shaped so that the flow becomes ever stronger. In such cases, we may become one of the streaming Serengeti-like multitudes charging along together in history's cohort, erasing the tracks of preceding generations; at some time becoming conscious of a new generation coming up behind us.

Without such organizing principals as generation, life would become an essentially aimless, timeless drifting from sensation to sensation, from experience to experience. Like the donkey between the carrot and the stick, we all too readily find ourselves seduced by an endless round of consumption, the point of which as Marcuse (1964) has pointed out, early in the study of consumer society, leaves us dissatisfied so that we continually need to consume more. Alternatively we are driven by work-priorities, surrounded by a battery of demands, seemingly without limit or obvious end. These activities fill our time to such an extent that our lives appear outside of time. We do not simply persist in time; however, we, as Small (2007) reminds us, age. Our adult identities change over time and, in many contemporary societies, this process is perceived negatively and is avoided. Taken together, these immediate experiences provide a powerful motivator not to look at generational identity. Until we stop and realize we are in a different place, and here the concern is a different place in the life course. It is this process of ageing that offers the life course pattern and purpose. And if there are patterns, the question arises of how they can be discovered in ourselves, and in seeing them cease to be immersed in their particular logic and reclaim some form of agency, of understanding, with respect to them.

The second area that requires an introductory explanation concerns two concepts that are very closely related, these being adult ageing and generations. Ageing happens to each individual throughout their life course, and while this is often thought of simply as a physical process, it is also a social one, determined by attitudes and expectations about behaviour. A distinctive way that age is related to generation, is through the passage of time, so that one is referred to as a member of the younger and older generation or as part of the millennium, IT, X, Y, boomer or war generation. These distinctions are often linked to particular historical experiences or change of affairs which offer persons born at a certain time a set of common reference points and social labels that help locate them in wider social space. The value of generation in the family sense is often evaluated through the lens of these common and distinguishing cohorts-driven, cultural and historical experiences. Family distinctions of generation are perhaps the most fluid, by degrees in terms of age and ageing. Becoming a parent or grandparent can happen across a range of chronological ages. One is, for the most part, born into a family at some point, yet one is also born into a social cohort which is then fixed and its labeling processes and iconic status travel with its members throughout their lives.

There are different levels in which age and generation impact on people's identities and position in society. Both concepts influence the way that we think and feel about intergenerational relations. That is to say our inner, imaginative worlds are already structured in generational terms, through individual experience, social development in families and through wider societal expectations and historical circumstances. We are aware of these influences by degrees, some consciously and some are unconscious. This inner world presents a liminal, fuzzy beginning to a journey towards generational understanding, where the influences of life-course experience, family lineage and historical cohort are often indistinct. Sometimes, it may be difficult to say where the boundary between inner and outer reality lies. We have memories and associations. Emotional echoes and ways of thinking that reach out to shape the world. It is not always easy to define where one begins and the other ends. At a different level, social expectations shape intergenerational relations in particular ways and form the stage on which thoughts and feelings are expressed or suppressed. Again these expectations are often unspoken and act as a sort of common sense which guide everyday behaviour and allow much of it to be taken for granted. However, this socially constructed reality is only one of many possible interpretations, even if it appears at times to be rigid and inflexible. In fact, attitudes to adult ageing and generational relations continue to change across cultures and in different historical periods. When these social realities are in transition; as they are when stable populations change their demographic shape, traditional attitudes and demands around adult ageing are challenged, the balance between state and privatized forms of care is threatened, or a new generational group or cohort challenges an existing social order: life becomes both more uncertain and more flexible. Thus changing age and generational relations present both a threat and an opportunity to actual intergenerational relationships, which can occur at the personal level, in social interaction, in institutions and organizations and in structural characteristics and imbalances of power.

The two concepts, age and generation come together in the notion of the 'age-other' someone who is constructed as being of a different group to oneself, based on age. Age-otherness may include aspects of life course and family position and cohort identity. Whether an individual is seen as being 'other' will be affected by the interaction of these elements of generational identity. So, in a certain social, cultural or historical context, a person of a certain chronological age may be labelled as being part of one category or another, such as being adolescent, middle-aged or very old. While in another, these would be categorized differently, or not at all. Similarly, the importance of family ties and generational positions may be more important than wider cohort group identities in one context, and less so in another. The importance given to family or periods in the individual life course, whether it is seen as a negative or positive source of identity may vary between historical cohorts cultural groups.

The distinctions outlined earlier have drawn attention to a third area of concern: the contexts within which age and generational relations are played out. Each has its effect on intergenerational relations in various areas including in families, in the workplace or in different community settings. It is argued that social, demographic, economic and cultural changes influence relations between generations and raise controversy, surrounding generational equity, inequality between generations and intergenerational justice (Lowenstein and Doron, 2008). At the time of writing, we know little, for example, about how increased life expectancy affects family members' interaction with older and younger kin; nor do we know how the perception that life is long affects decisions about investments in children and grandchildren and expectations in each generation about providing and receiving help at different life stages (Hagestad, 2003). Certain issues may be raised in this regard, however: further studying the features of family, work, social policy initiatives as institutions that coordinate the sometimes competing goals of individuals or groups. Examining if families have particular ways of resolving conflicts may be one way of judging the relative benefit of family membership as compared to other social groups. Looking at sources of generational solidarity and the differences across various social and cultural contexts; looking at the benefits and costs of group membership, how it is distributed within and between generations, and what explains inequality between generations. Trying to understand if norms generated by social and economic context affect choices and the process by which generations in a variety of contexts make choices and negotiate relationships.

Given the temporal nature of ageing and of generational progression, intergenerational relations need to be understood by including a life-course approach and taking life transitions into account (Rossi and Rossi, 1990), empirical evidence show that parents and children differ qualitatively in the ways in which they relate to one another, the way they negotiate relationships over time and especially as frailty sets in for older parents as each generation experiences such life transition differently.

We would argue, in this regard, that sustainable intergenerational relationships will need to rely on increased levels of generational insight, empathy and mutually negotiated action which might be especially needed during life transitions.

Intelligence of this sort facilitates the interplay between different levels of understanding associated with intergenerational exchanges. Such deeper understanding should allow us to move beyond varying conceptual positions, such as family or cohort and macro or micro, obligation or choice, which can give credence to inflexible responses to related social issues. An intelligent approach to intergenerational relations would need to address the issue of how individuals become self-consciously aware of their generational status, and thereby encounter and under optimal conditions be able to put themselves in the position of the age-other.

How far these processes influence the experience of and action towards others in the social world would largely depend on the relative ability to act with awareness of one's own generational circumstances. This would be activated by the ability to reflect and act, which draws on an understanding of one's own life course, family and social history, placed within a contemporary social climate.

Structure of the book

This book offers a new conceptual approach to the study of intergenerational relations from various disciplinary perspectives, relating to the individual, family and social levels of analysis. The introduction paints the rationale and background and sets the context for the book. Thereafter, the first chapter gives an exposition of Generational Intelligence and broad views on what it is, presenting the steps one has to undergo to eventually achieve a higher level. The next two chapters deal with self-awareness, focusing on the internal world of the imagination, and discussing the various paths towards achieving Generational Intelligence. It is followed by two chapters on the self and others – emphasizing the impact of social ageism and other phenomena on generational strategies, negotiating ambivalence and using masquerade to create critical spaces for intergenerational engagement.

The second part of the book, which includes five chapters, focuses on specific areas where intergenerational relations are played out: Generational Intelligence in families, in caregiving, in relation to elder abuse, in the workplace and in community programmes. Each of these chapters begins with an introduction to the topic and a review of the relevant literature. Each chapter then continues with a novel conceptualization of Generational Intelligence and its implications for the relevant topic discussed in the chapter. The last concluding chapter discusses sustainability – the possibility of negotiating relations over time and strengthening ones that last.

This book begins to map out some of the key issues, paradoxes and contradictions in the study of intergenerational relationships today and in the future. We introduced an innovative conceptual framework for understanding and action which we hope will engage the readers and act as an impetus for further critical thinking in this area. It should add impetus to what we already know or want to discover. As social scientists we face the challenge of explaining how intergenerational relations are acted and negotiated by the individual, within families and in broader social contexts, how these processes unfold and what do they entail. Our work grew out of our quest for explanations and understanding of issues of intergenerational relations and critically looking at existing theoretical perspectives. We hope the development and formulation of the new concept of Generational Intelligence will be a further step in this direction.

Note

1 OASIS (Old Age and Autonomy: The Role of Service Systems and Intergenerational Family Solidarity) was funded by the EU under the fifth framework programme.

1   What is Generational Intelligence?

Summary

The purpose of this chapter is to draw out a newly emerging model of intergenerational relationships, called Generational Intelligence. It takes as its starting point the degree to which it is possible to place oneself in the position of a person of a different age or in what has been designated as a different generation. In it, we explore an approach that is based on how generations are experienced as part of everyday social life. A point we make is, that in a time of changing roles and expectations it is important to re-focus attention to the processes that underpin these kinds of relationships. To this end, a working distinction is made between the informational 'intelligence' that is culturally available to social actors and the degree to which it is possible to think and act 'intelligently' within that defining context. This is followed by four steps that someone would need to take to become critically aware of age and generational identity as a factor in social relationships. The steps include a growing awareness of oneself as being influenced by age and generation, so that in the end it is possible to recognize one's personal generational distinctiveness. Other steps follow from this, such as understanding other people based on similarities and differences between generations, becoming critically aware of the values underlying social assumptions about generations and adult ageing and finally, acting in a manner that is generationally aware. In this manner, we work towards an understanding of two key aspects of intergenerational relations. First, the degree to which it is possible to place oneself in the position of the age-other and second, the possibility of working towards negotiated and sustainable solutions.

Key points

- In everyday life, generation is taken for granted, experienced holistically and is not necessarily actively thought about.
- To make sense of it a critical distance has to be created, by becoming consciously aware of one's own generational identity.

- As part of this process, it is necessary to separate and then return to the 'age-other' so that the distinctiveness of each position can be recognized.
- This process involves becoming critically aware of the values and attitudes underpinning beliefs about intergenerational relations.
- The process clears the way for action that is generationally sustainable.

Introduction

This chapter is grounded on two questions which are followed up in subsequent parts of the book. First, how can we put ourselves in the place of someone of another generation? And, second, how is it possible to negotiate intergenerationally sustainable solutions? The first of these is necessary because, in life-course terms, contemporary society so often eclipses the existential projects of the second half of adult life and replaces them with the priorities of the first. This seems at first glance to make putting oneself into the shoes of the age-other an easy task. In effect, to the person in the dominant stage, their goals, hopes, desires and sense of past and future, appear to be universally acknowledged. On closer inspection, however, the task becomes a considerable psychological and social challenge. The second is necessary because it is not simply enough to become self-consciously aware of one's own and another's life-course priorities. It is also important to achieve a rapport between them, and find ways of negotiating a complementary relationship that can be sustained over time. It has, in other words to work for both parties and to be able to last.

As a starting point, it may be helpful to put forward a preliminary definition. We would define Generational Intelligence as an ability to reflect and act, which draws on an understanding of one's own and others' life-course, family and social history, placed within its social and cultural context.

Intergenerational relations provide the context within which individuals grow and mature. They provide the backdrop against which people mark their own ageing and the value that is attached to that process. Their quality shapes the way we feel, think and act towards others.

Generational Intelligence not only focuses on a single person's or generations' perspective but also creates the possibility of a space emerging, in which multiple generational viewpoints can be taken into account. This gives the opportunity for a process of pragmatic negotiation to take place. It arises as people become explicitly aware of similarities and differences based on age. If age groups do not aim to occupy the same social position within this space, complementary processes based on age-distinctiveness and solidarity may be able to emerge. It does not suggest an 'age-neutral' or 'age-irrelevant' society, however, but the negotiation of generation-specific needs and goals.

Generational relations as a growing social issue

How, then, can we put ourselves in the position of someone of a different age group? How far is it possible to understand the different influences on intergenerational activity? How far can we act while taking them into account? These are key questions for the twenty-first century as the numbers of older citizens are growing to equal those of children and adults in midlife (Bengtson and Lowenstein, 2003). People are living longer, with changes in age structure affecting both the developed and developing worlds (Aboderin, 2004). The proportional growth of the number of older adults and the length of time that people are living is historically unprecedented (WHO, 2000). As a result, we are increasingly living in a world where challenges to existing assumptions and expectations about intergenerational behaviour can be expected (Biggs *et al.*, 2011). The higher life-expectancy of older persons is already creating new spaces for multigenerational interaction, as there are simply more generations to interact with each other (Antonucci *et al.*, 2001) to which can be added an increased complexity of extended family patterns arising from divorce, remarriage and other forms of relationships (Bengtson *et al.*, 2003). Individuals may be living in the context of four or in some cases five generations, in circumstances where kin relations are becoming more diverse.

In addition to these demographic shifts, a new range of social issues are emerging, that are intergenerational in form. These include age discrimination in the workplace, elder abuse in care, questions of generational fairness around pensions and whether healthcare should be rationed according to age. Such issues have been recognized by the Second World Assembly on Ageing in Madrid, convened by the UN in 2002, which noted: 'the need to strengthen solidarity between generations and intergenerational partnerships, keeping in mind the particular needs of both older and younger ones, and encourage mutually responsive relationships between generations' (UN, 2002b: 4).

This is not only a problem of numbers, however. It is also a problem of developing the intellectual and cultural capacity for societies to adapt to this situation. Generation itself, has been referred to as a 'packed social concept' (McDaniel, 2008), including a variety of social, familial and personal associations, that influence personal identity. Unfortunately the different disciplines which are engaged with the concept of generation, such as sociology, psychology, medicine, geography, rarely cross-communicate (Bengtson and Lowenstein, 2003). Each emphasizes a particular perspective and struggles to deliver an understanding of how a multiplicity of different influences contributes to the ways people navigate their social world. Partly as a result of the aforementioned, there is a growing recognition that to study adult ageing one has also to study intergenerational relationships (Antonucci *et al.*, 2007). Intergenerational relations provide the context within which individuals grow and change, the way that they mark their own ageing and the relative value that is attached to that process.

Taken together, these factors point to a need to re-examine the idea of generation, its constituent parts and how it is experienced. What follows is an attempt at unwrapping what an increasing critical awareness of generation might entail, in other words, what forms of 'intelligence' are required to understand and act in the context of other generations. By critical, here, is meant an ability to see beyond the surface assumptions that drive everyday behaviour, address power relations between generational groups, plus a valuing of the experiential element of ageing and encounters between age groups. It has been assumed that age categories, such as midlife, old age and adolescence cannot easily be given specific chronological ages (Jung, 1931; Shweder, 1998; Schaie and Willis, 2002; Settersten, 2006). They depend, for example, upon particular functional capacities and how ageing is perceived in any society. Similarly, generations are often more likely to be a combination of social Labeling and self-perception. The degree to which an individual sees themselves as a member of a group based on age and different from other age groups, or age-others, does not depend on breaking the population down into demographically convenient ten-year chunks, but on how that generation is socially constructed and experienced.

Generations, power and cultural resources

The need to interrogate different degrees of Generational Intelligence is made more pressing in the light of comments by contemporary social theorists. For example, Kohli has argued that 'in the twenty-first century, the class conflict seems to be defunct and its place taken over by the generational conflict' (2005: 518). This assertion gains some support from Turner (1998) who has outlined generational tension between baby boomers and younger generations on the distribution of power. Francophone writers such as Ricard (Olazabal, 2005) and Chauvel (2007a) have criticized the boomer or generation lyric for social self-ishness and disproportionate cultural and economic influence, to the disadvantage of succeeding generational groups. Moody (2008) has charted what he calls the 'boomer wars' as a recurrent polarization of discourse in North American popular literature, while in UK politics, Willetts (2010) has blamed the boomer generation for using up resources belonging to other generational groups. Conflict and competition in the public sphere of policy, work and popular debate, may be expected to increase the salience of generational similarity and difference. This is in spite of evidence that indicates that, at least in the private sphere, generational transfers continue to travel downward, from older to younger generations (Irwin, 1998) and that family solidarity exists across systems that rely on family or state-based welfare support (Daatland and Lowenstein, 2005; Daatland *et al.*, 2010).

Social commentaries, especially those arising from the public sphere, then, suggest a renewed aggression in intergenerational discourse, directed primarily against late-midlife intergenerational relations. Indeed, a number of social problems are likely to multiply as populations live longer, and the proportion of older adults increases. If it is accepted that increased scarcity of resources, leads to a retrenchment into in-group identification, and that identities are increasingly being cast in terms of generation, obscuring other forms of social inequality, then the degree to which it is possible to put oneself in the position of someone of a different age group may become one of the defining factors driving social policy in the twenty-first century.

Our collective ability to deal with the issues thrown up by an ageing population will only be as good as the cultural tools available to us. This is not only a problem of numbers, however. It is also a problem of developing the intellectual and cultural capacity for societies to adapt to this situation. The cultural processes that have been available to date, reflect attempts either to ensure continuity of social value in terms defined by a dominant age group or of the transfer of power from one generation to the next. Older adults may, for example, continue to be encouraged to remain as productive workers, either paid or unpaid (Morrow-Howell *et al.*, 2001), or they may find a role as consumers (Gilleard and Higgs, 2005), thus in one way or another feeding wider economic interests. These positions have now largely replaced attempts to ease a path of disengagement or of unspecified, yet morally signified activity (Katz, 2000; Estes *et al.*, 2003). Disengagement refers to a withdrawal from social participation and a restriction in social roles in order to make room for succeeding generations. Activity, here, refers to the need for older people to 'stay active', but without necessarily identifying its purpose.

One implication of a transformation in expectations of later life is that a new architecture for social relations may begin to emerge. Should anyone doubt the dramatic change that has occurred in attitudes to later life, for example, it is only necessary to compare two statements, 20 years apart, made by the United Nations. The First World Assembly on ageing (1982) concluded that:

> The human race is characterized by a long childhood and a long old age. Throughout history this has enabled older persons to educate the younger and pass on values to them. . . . A longer life provides humans with an opportunity to examine their lives in retrospect, to correct some of their mistakes, to get closer to the truth and to achieve a different understanding of the sense and value of their actions.
>
> (United Nations, 1982: 1b)

This can be seen in retrospect to illustrate a rather gentle view of generational relations and the tasks of ageing, with an emphasis on retrospection, wisdom and a sense of summing up. A sort of benign disengagement.

While demographic projections remained essentially the same, in 2002, the Second World Assembly on Ageing, showed a very different vision of later life.

> The potential of older persons is a powerful basis for future development. This enables society to rely increasingly on the skills, experience and wisdom of older persons, not only to take the lead in their own betterment but also to participate actively in that society as a whole.
>
> (United Nations, 2002: 2)

The first statement suggests a personal task looking backwards and sifting through accrued experience. The second privileges the application of skills in the here and now, while looking forward. By 2002, there seem to be fewer qualities that distinguish one generation from another and less emphasis on specifically inter-generational relations. However intergenerational relations continue to provide the context within which individuals age, the way that they mark their own ageing and the relative value that is attached to that process. It is becoming clear that we do not currently, as national or global societies, have the cultural resources, the redundant cultural strength, to draw on to negotiate this novel intergenerational situation. We are, collectively, rather like midlifers who, according to Dan McAdams (1985), have to 'figure it out on their own'. Traditional roles and responsibilities no longer seem to fit and the new demands lack the specificity and cultural embeddedness to supply a reliable guide to action.

Towards a phenomenology of generation

A key beginning for Generational Intelligence is to recognize that while the scientific study of population ageing uses separate categories, such as historical period, cohorts within a certain age-range, family position or stage of life, it is rarely encountered in such an atomized way during daily interaction. Rather, we would argue, generational identity is experienced as an undifferentiated whole, all in one go, as part of who one is. While the salience of different influences would vary with context and circumstance; generation, as an amalgam of life-stage, family position and cultural labeling, is generally experienced as a felt degree of similarity or distance with respect to others loosely based on something to do with age.

Arber and Attias-Donfut (2000) have observed that a feeling of generational belonging is created not just in a horizontal dimension of the birth cohort but also in a vertical dimension of familial lineage and that questions of generational awareness exist at the intersection of these axes. To this can be added Biggs' (1999) distinction between depth and surface elements of life-course experience, dimensions of the mature self which creates a third context, that of the maturation of personal consciousness. This third context is perhaps more difficult to explore empirically, and exists tacitly as a growing awareness of one's progress through life and the existential tensions that emerge as a result. This meeting point of birth cohort, familial lineage and personal maturation creates a three-dimensional space in which the immediate experience of generational identity, its phenomenology, exists and is given holistic expression. It is the quality and critical consciousness of this space that informs behaviour in intergenerational settings. The thoughts, feelings and values associated with that space, the degree to which people are aware of it, how they react to it, the effect it has on the sense of who they are and how they behave towards others form a basis for what might be called 'Generational Intelligence'.

By choosing a critical phenomenological form of inquiry, we recognize, then, that while each dimension may be conceptually discrete, they are experienced holistically and it is their sum or balance which results in a particular experience of generation. Becoming conscious of one's own distinctive identity emerges as a force that both links and distinguishes particular generational groups in so far as it is not until one becomes conscious of generational distinctiveness that one can develop genuine relationships between generations (Faimberg, 2005). So, consciousness of generation, may depend upon being able both to recognize one's own generational identity and how that identity itself generates certain forms of relationship. The point here is not simply to rehearse the observation that adult demography consists of cohort, period and lifespan effects, but also to suggest that generation is experienced as a combination of influences, experienced as a whole, which give it its individual phenomenological flavour. In order to critically interrogate this experiential space, an individual needs to separate out competing influences, and consciously return to them before genuine intergenerational understanding can emerge. Such influences should be thought of processes, which come in and out of focus at different times.

Linking generation and experience

An understanding of generations, when we think about it at all, is, then, mediated by other experiences such as that of the family, one's current position in the life-course and whether one's age group has shared historical events that become socially signified. There are a number of research reports indicating that different notions of generation are closely linked and exist at the crossroads of public and private experience.

Hagestad (2003) has observed that families often mediate between individuals and societies undergoing change, while much of Bengtson's (2001) work has concentrated on the family as a place where the influence of relationships and social structures meet. Here, intergenerational relations within families represent complex social bonds, and family members are linked by multiple types of relationship that may produce solidarity, conflictual or ambivalent feelings (Luescher and Pillemer, 1998; Pillemer *et al.*, 2007). Bengtson and Putney (2006) claim that intergenerational relations within multigenerational families have a profound but unrecognized influence on relations between age groups at the societal level.

Perhaps, the most widely known evidence of the relationship between generations and historical and economic circumstances can be found in the work of Elder (1974; 1994), whose longitudinal study of life chances following the Great Depression and economic downturn in the North American Midwest, links the three metrics of individual lifetime, family time and historical time. The linkage between particular ages and family events and historical circumstances shows that the character taken by certain generations depends on broad social changes like migration, wars or economic shifts, which shape mutual support within families (Hareven, 1996; Elder, 1980). Position in the family, age at which economic hardship is experienced and gender were each found to mediate life chances and certain aspects of personality. In France, Attias-Donfut (2003; Attias-Donfut and Wolff, 2005) has addressed generational interdependence in families as mitigating the effects of 'discontinuity of social destinies'. Attias-Donfut's work has focused on cultural transmission and generational memories and as such, constitutes a powerful attempt to place the protective role of families within a social and historical context. The cohort one is born into, she states, shapes one's personal destiny, through prevailing social conditions 'At the time of entry into professional life, notably concerning the educational system and the labour market' (2003: 214). In the French postwar context at least three socio-historical phases can be identified, which she calls the generation of labour, of abundance and of under-protection. Successive cohorts, therefore, do not have the same life chances. Family and kinship ties, which are themselves subject to multigenerational changes in fortune, can nevertheless protect family members through generational interdependence, and can subvert official versions of events by preserving and transmitting their own oral histories. The memory of historical events is itself shaped by the role of family members in passing the experience of social events on to younger generations, as 'each generation has one foot in the history which formed its predecessor and one in its own history and time' (Attias-Donfut and Wolff, 2005: 453).

The work of Elder, Attias-Donfut and their associates demonstrates that the protective role of the family can be uneven and equivocal and can only be understood in close relationship to an individual's life stage and to cohort histories. Experience rests on a combination of generational influences.

The combined influence of different factors associated with generation and holistic experience, may help explain the increasing popularity of seeing generations in terms of their habitus (Turner, 1998; Gilleard and Higgs, 2005). Habitus is a term arising from the work of Bourdieu (1979), the French social philosopher, to describe a sort of social space containing particular lifestyles and cultural attitudes. If generation can be thought of as a space one can enter, it can be freed from associations with a fixed age group and allows generational identity to be seen much more in terms of a lifestyle choice. Thus, Gilleard (2004) has argued that generation can be thought of as a distinct yet temporally located cultural phenomenon within which individuals from a potential variety of overlapping birth cohorts can participate. Gilleard further points out that generational styles of consciousness arising from a specific 'habitus', both generate and structure an individual's behaviour and self-perception. Gilleard and Higgs (2005), therefore, talk about the blurring of generational differences, and the creation of cohort-based 'cultures of ageing'. Further, a number of writers have argued that generational difference reflects existential questions concerning passage through the human life-course itself. Differences occur as a consequence of increased recognition that life is finite, changing life-projects between early and late adulthood and that forms of social engagement and insight vary with increasing age (Dittman-Kohli, 1990; 2005; Biggs, 1999; Westerhof and Barrett, 2005) the common point of reference of both habitus and life-projects is that both make an identified generation contingent upon experience. It is no longer fixed by age or lineage, but adopts the qualities of a strategy or chosen identity.

When the study of familial, life-course and social cohort-based generations is compared, one can see a move away from formal relations towards an understanding of generations based on personal or collective experience and self-conscious identities. If, as has been argued elsewhere, 'generation' is a crossroads phenomenon, where a number of social influences intersect (Biggs, 2007), then it is not unreasonable to begin to explore the phenomenology of that experience and the processes that might make one factor more salient than others, or individuals more or less willing to use generation as a self-conscious form of engagement with the world.

A phenomenology of generational awareness

Our argument begins from the observation that generation is experienced in imme-diate action as a phenomenological whole. Even though it may arise from attitudes to life-course, family or cohort, experientially speaking, these are secondary con-structs. For example, when UK baby boomers were asked about their generational experience, they responded holistically, drawing intuitively on different aspects of generation as it is used in common understanding and moving freely between and combining demographic categories (Biggs *et al.*, 2007). Generation, in this sense as a phenomenological unity corresponds to what Bollas (1991) refers to as a simple, or immersive, state of mind. Unless certain disconfirming events throw individuals out of this immersion in the everydayness of life, 'generation' is used but rarely reflected upon. Bollas argues that, with age, adults become increasingly aware that their generational identity is no longer at the cultural centre, and as such it becomes subject to critical self-awareness. With an increasingly sophisticated perspective, concepts common in the literature, describing conflict solidarity and ambivalence, each referring to life-course, lineage or cohort contexts, are less use-ful as typologies, or mutually exclusive categories. Rather, they should be thought of as phenomenological positions arising from the differential emphasis placed upon them. And, as they become the subject of critical awareness, become strate-gies that are adopted towards intergenerational relationships, rather than embed-ded characteristics. Accordingly, while generation is immersively experienced all in one go, it may be actively strategized as arising from one position or another.

In terms of life-categories an individual may, in life-course terms be in midlife, in family terms be part of a sandwiched generation and belong to the baby-boomer cohort. As a phenomenological space, she or he may change from looking back to reference points in childhood, to looking forward to the amount of time they think they might have left, wondering how competing family demands will allow them to use this time to best advantage, identifying with younger rather than older generations, and striving for self-actualization. Their awareness of self and others is generationally inflected and an amalgam of influences which have yet to be des-ignated or understood, but nevertheless affects intergenerational behaviour, even if it is not always being thought about.

Degrees of Generational Intelligence would influence self-conscious aware-ness of such generational positioning and how far 'generation' is recognized in the experience of the social world. Individuals have varying degrees of access to this material, depending on their exposure to facilitative contexts. These contexts would allow the more deeply immersed elements of past experience and contem-porary meaning to emerge into consciousness (Biggs, 1999). The journey from immersion, to a recognition of different influences, which may be strategized or recombined into a complex whole, form the basis for generationally intelligent action.

What is Generational Intelligence?

Becoming aware of generational perspectives

In outlining a model, that has been given the working name of 'Generational Intelligence', an attempt has been made to plot the process by which individuals or groups are made capable of seeing from alternative age-perspectives. The question being posed is what sort of 'intelligence' might be needed to engage with the age-other within a generationally inflected space.

As such, the processes identified would apply to any age group, constituted as different from another in the eyes of at least one group. Identifying another person as being of a different age, an age-other, is not a quantifiable difference when speaking about Generational Intelligence, but is rather phenomenologically real in the sense that a difference is perceived to exist by one or both of the actors involved. This difference may be based on cohort differences, such as that between the 'baby-boomers' and their parents (Phillipson *et al.*, 2008) or the 'IT' generation and age groups who are less ICT literate (Edmunds and Turner, 2005). It may be based on lineage within families, where a different generational position is biologically and socially visible (Bengtson and Lowenstein, 2003). It may also result from the occupation of a different phase of life, such as for example, adolescence or childhood, or the first decades of adulthood or midlife (Biggs, 1999). In each case, a difference based on age is socially signified and acts to guide the way in which each actor constructs a sense of self and of those who are age-others. Because such a difference is thereby socially real, it becomes a barrier to mutual understanding that then has to be overcome. The endpoint would be an ability to act knowingly within an intergenerational space, so that thinking, feeling and behaviour take a critical understanding of generation into account. Because the label 'generation', as an amalgam of life-course, cohort and family is somewhat protean in everyday experience, we have tended to use the phrase 'age-other' to refer to identities that emerge based on generational location, rather than identify particular ages or time periods that hold a specific generation in place. The visibility of a particular aspect would depend on context, as does the type of age-otherness that is most salient.

In terms of age similarity, the notion of an age-other points towards at least two types. On the one hand, there is what might be called 'simple similarity'. This is when no barrier exists in the socially constructed realities of either party with respect to age identity. Complex similarity, however, has a deeper structure in so far as age difference has at first been recognized and is then denied. In this sense, it might exist as what Bollas (1987) has called an 'unthought known'. An unthought known has been suppressed from phenomenological experience, but is nevertheless present as a guiding principle for everyday activity. It rests on the idea that in order to suppress something, to hide it so to speak from everyday expression, it had to have at some point been recognized. While Bollas was largely speaking about unconscious processes, it is also possible to see interpersonal activities such as masquerade (Biggs, 1999) as means of acting on the basis of something that is hidden and may also be hidden from the actor themselves.

Once an age-other has been identified, the question of how one relates to them becomes an issue. How does one evaluate the relationship, does it occasion rivalry and conflict, solidarity and common cause, or mixed feelings? Mixed feelings suggest a more complex position in which the actors recognize ambivalence. Rather than wholeheartedly and probably unreflectively liking or disliking the age-other, both emotions need to be dealt with within the same space.

The move beyond single positions while keeping alternative generational perspectives simultaneously in mind moves the intergenerational terrain on from conflict, towards a consideration of how one can live with the ambivalence that inevitably arises. If some theoretical positions argue that there is more conflict than harmony, while others that there is more harmony than conflict, a generationally intelligent position would recognize that there is both harmony and conflict. Creating a critical distance between different potential positions, gives room to manoeuvre and reflect. One no longer acts out a single position rather one acts with them and is able to strategize around alternatives previously expressed as being in opposition or mutually incompatible. One is no longer caught in their grip.

Deploying Generational Intelligence

There's intelligence and intelligence

It might be useful at this point to make a distinction between two ways of using the term 'intelligence'. One refers to forms of information or everyday data that are culturally available and can be collected in order to make sense of the world. In generational terms, this may include the expectations held about generationally related behavior and the cultural shortcuts used, both tacitly and explicitly, to make sense of age and generational distinctions. In other words, we gather intelligence about age and generation as a guide to appropriate conduct. The second use lies in working 'intelligently' with such data. This would involve a way of seeing through generationally tinted glasses, a way of interpreting the world, to draw out how social reality has been generationally constructed. This second use of intelligence would pay attention to the degree to which actors and groups behave as if they are immersed in their own group-specific form of generational consciousness or are able to use more complex forms that include multiple generational perspectives. So, at an everyday level, Generational Intelligence can refer to the forms of information that are available to the active subject, in the sense of the 'intelligence' current in any one situation. Rather like the way that spies use the phrase to discriminate available and potentially available clues, Generational Intelligence refers to a seeking out information, a search for data. Here it is helpful to distinguish between information that is available within any one social or cultural context, the degree to which the social actor is aware of these sources and the extent to which they are used to make sense of the age-other. The second use lies in working 'intelligently' with such raw material, evaluating the source and discerning what has not been said. Generational Intelligence, in this sense, denotes different degrees to which social actors behave reflexively with respect to generational identities and intergenerational relations. Such a reflexive awareness of generation creates room for manoeuvre. It creates a distance between immersion inside a generational identity and being able to step outside in order to take a position with respect to the generational identities that are available. It turns fixed positions into options.

Outlining the dimensions of Generational Intelligence

Generational Intelligence consists of certain dimensions, which include degrees of self-awareness, a capacity for intergenerational empathy and an ability to act in a generationally aware manner.

As a starting point in the study of generational experience, it is important to ask about the degree to which one becomes conscious of oneself as part of a generation. It is quite possible to continue through adult life without actively using generational categories to guide social understanding. While we are aware of generational distinctions in the wider environment, they may be submerged in Berger and Luckman's (1976) common sense experience or have become what Bollas (1987) calls part of an 'unthought known'. However, in order not simply to act out these un-thought-about determinants, to be self-consciously aware of them in order to understand and control their influence, it is important to recognize them. Recognizing generation as an issue is the pragmatic equivalent of the philosophical task involved in determining degrees of generational awareness. Once generational positions are recognized as influencing personal identity and behaviour, it is possible to identify how one's own position differs from others. Generation, in other words, becomes intergenerational.

Once social actors become conscious of themselves as part of a generation; as a parent, as a member of the 'war generation' as being in 'adolescence'; the relative ability to put themselves in the position of other generations also becomes an issue. At least when it comes to personal ageing, there is a growing body of evidence, arising from Jung's (1931) original distinction between 'first and second halves of life', that there are significant discontinuities between different parts of adult life as it is experienced (Tornstam, 2005; Dittmann-Kohli, 2005). These discontinuities arise from a differential awareness of personal finitude and changed existential priorities as adults grow older and contribute to a sense of generational distinctiveness.

If one lives, however, as if there are no generational distinctions, as if everyone were the same in terms of this temporal classification, then there would be no reason to see another person as belonging to a different or similar generational group. One might assume, as many of the UK boomers claimed to do, that there was essentially no difference in identity between themselves and their adult children (Biggs *et al.*, 2007). They conformed to the view that age-distinctions were becoming increasingly blurred (Hepworth, 2004; Gilleard and Higgs, 2005). It is important to distinguish this way of thinking from being unaware of generational distinction, as here distinctions are consciously recognized as the first step in denying their influence. A perspective that denies difference may create certain disadvantages if age-related changes are ignored, while they continue to influence behaviour and social attitudes; for example, in situations where different age groups were expected to compete, at work, in sports, as consumers of services, on equal terms without taking their particular attributes into account (Biggs, 2005). In such cases, generational attributes represent both cultural and life-course related phenomena. They can be ascribed as well as achieved and generational identities may arise from personal experience or from social expectation. They may vary in salience depending upon context or historical period. Each will influence the degree to which it is desirable or even possible to see the world as it is seen from a different age or generational position. An ability to place oneself in the position of the age-other would depend upon the readiness of mass media and cultural trends to identify alternative age perspectives, on public policies that facilitate the expression of age-specific skills and competencies and on interpersonal behaviour that valued complimentarity rather than similarity as a basis for social exchange.

The pragmatic equivalent of this dimension would be the degree to which it is possible to negotiate intergenerational consensus. The UK boomers would need to ask their children whether they thought that the generational groupings had become blurred, on what dimensions and with what effect, for example. Helping professionals and even social researchers would need to negotiate between generational groups and their concerns and be aware that their own generational position influences the way that outcomes are achieved. Policy-makers would need to distinguish between their projected desire to live a certain way in later life, based on their current age identity, and the perspectives of individuals in deep old age.

Once one has become self-aware of a personal generational identity and become sensitized to distinctions between self and other on the basis of generational attributes, the question arises of a relative ability to act with awareness of one's generational circumstances. Here, we would need to know much more about how this dimension works and the ways that generationally informed decisions are made. It is possible, and probably most common, for example, for social actors to be aware of their own generational identity, recognize the differences between this and other age-related positions and nevertheless discount the latter in preference of the former when it comes to deciding on a course of action. In certain positions of authority, such as in the helping professions there may be codes that regulate intergenerational behaviour, such as in child-care or elder-care. The midlife boomer described earlier may experience tension between the cultural-generational marker of self-actualization and the social expectation to care for a parent who perhaps has not, in life-course terms, been facilitative of that development. The pragmatic question that this dimension highlights would be the degree to which people are able to act on mutually productive solutions.

These three dimensions of Generational Intelligence raise some basic questions that have not been at the forefront of the debate on generational consciousness in families and societies. Such questions would include: what each individual brings into the intergenerational familial and societal exchange. How conscious they are of what they bring. How relations are performed and negotiated within the encounter. The degree of impact had on the process, outcome and potential for connection, conflict or ambivalence, between generations. Whether it builds capacity for understanding different generations and their needs?

Steps towards Generational Intelligence

This combination of a complex generational self that is reflected on as an object, a recognition of balance and imbalance and the construction of a social reality that makes available certain templates for generational identities, contributes to the salience and deployment of Generational Intelligence.

If Generational Intelligence is unevenly distributed, in terms of generations and age groups, then it follows that there are certain steps that might exist, taking social actors from one state of awareness to another. It also suggests certain processes that would need to occur, in order to establish higher degrees of generational sensitivity. It can, perhaps, be broken down into identifiable steps that are liable to increase the likelihood of generationally intelligent understanding and action. By taking such steps, immediate experience can follow pathways into more complex and reflective processes. It involves a process of separation and return which allows a critical reflective space to emerge. As this space is entered, it provokes recognition of the relationship between self and other that leads to further action taking place beyond immersion. These steps might look like this:

Step One: self-exploration and generational awareness. This would be necessary in order to locate oneself within generational space and to identify different contributory factors that are expressed through generational identity. It involves an exploration of the inner world of generation, its imaginative contents and processes. The degree to which one's immediate phenomenology is affected by cohort, family and life- course position would need to be critically interrogated. Socio-historical attitudes to family influences thoughts and feelings, about oneself as a child, parent and grandparent, how progress through a person's own life-course affects attitudes, towards adolescence, the child-rearing years, and folds back into cohort identities would need to be disaggregated and understood. This may be primarily an interior process where parts of a holistic, yet immersive awareness of self are separated out prior to being returned to as a self-consciously aware whole. It is, as a first footfall, necessary to become aware that generational distinctiveness actually exists. This is a rather obvious point to make were it not for the tendency for certain policy statements (Biggs *et al.*, 2007) and identity positions (Biggs *et al.*, 2007) to deny or obscure it. Recognizing distinctiveness would be necessary in order to locate oneself within generational space and to identify different contributory factors that are expressed through generational identity. The degree to which one's immediate experience is affected by cohort, family and life-course position would need to be critically interrogated as part of this process. Socio-historical attitudes to family, for example, will influence a person's thoughts and feelings about themselves as a child, parent and grandparent, and progress through their own life-course as one phase leads on to another from adolescence, through to midlife and on into old age. How these distinctions fold back into cohort identities would need to be disaggregated and understood. At this point self-awareness, would be principally a personal reflective endeavour, an interior process where immersive awareness is separated out and made the subject of conscious reflection.

Step Two: understanding the relationship between generational positions. This examines the relationship between self and other, based on age and generation. The purpose of this second step would be to identify the key generational actors in any one situation and develop a generationally sensitized perspective, thus making intergenerational relations explicit. Generational relations include the positions that each social actor may hold, but also the associations that each person brings with them about other generations, their internal and external sets of representations that are organized generationally. This may include influences based on the experience of family, the cultural assumptions of different historical cohorts and the existential life-tasks that an individual currently faces. As part of this process, it would be possible to see the age-other as a person with priorities, desires, fears and reflections that may or may not overlap with one's own, thus engaging with the difficult tasks of placing oneself in the position of that age-other. Generational Intelligence would thereby begin a process that moves beyond binary thinking, such as identifying exclusively with either conflict or solidarity, while recognizing that age-based relations are based on multiple perspectives.

Step Three: taking a value stance towards generational positions. Knowing that generational distinctiveness and difference exist is no guarantee of the quality of the relations that emerge. It is quite possible that participants in generational exchange take an antagonistic position, one based on harmony, on mixed feelings or on indifference. Each of these suggests a value position supported by certain power relations, and as Generational Intelligence's own value position is one of increasing the likelihood of harmonious accommodation between generations, being explicit about the position taken is important at this stage. Rather than assume that actions concerning generational relations are in themselves neutral or objective, the task would be to critically assess the relations that tacitly and explicitly underpin intergenerational behavior. This is part of finding the ground on which we stand, which for critical gerontologists would require examination of generational power and how it might be negotiated. Therefore it is necessary to introduce a moral dimension at this stage, which may create different problems for social scientists, advocates and helping professionals to critically assess the values that tacitly and explicitly underpin intergenerational behaviour. Values that is, in Taylor's (1989) sense, that in the process of becoming self-aware, we need to commit to a place on which we will make our stand. So, for example, rather than simply assume that older adults should withdraw from society, or remain actively engaged, it is important to consider the assumptions driving these expectations, to what degree they are good or bad and why.

Step Four: concerns action, in a manner that is generationally aware. Once a value stance has been identified with respect to differences in generational power, the ground on which action can take place is made much clearer. The contributory element to this process would be the discovery of spaces that allow critical distance to emerge between competing positions. This would form the basis for informed strategies to emerge between generations. The value stance driving such activity would be to achieve sustainable partnerships that will be lasting and adaptive to changing circumstances. Generationally intelligent action would take place in the knowledge of one's own contribution and those of others and in the service of negotiated solutions. Action would work towards situations that move from immersion towards active accommodations between participants in the intergenerational encounter, as it is in this way that generational relationships might emerge that can stand the test of time. As part of this process, critical spaces are created that allow comparison and questioning of established activities. Keeping alternative generational perspectives simultaneously in mind moves the intergenerational terrain on from fixed positions, towards a consideration of how one can flexibly encounter the perspective of the age-other and act on it. It raises the possibility that intergenerational relations can be negotiated and sustained.

Taken together, these stages lead to a way of seeing through a generationally sensitized lens, in order to draw out how social reality has been generationally inflected and how sustainable negotiation around resources might take place. It is important, however, to engage in such a process without falling into the trap of saying what old age or other phases of adult ageing should be like. Rather, the objective would be to make a preliminary sketch of the processes that might have to take place to allow sustainable solutions to emerge, where sustainability refers to negotiations that take differing generational perspectives and requirements into account.

Mapping generational encounters

The four steps outlined above might also be used to facilitate the mapping of particular generational encounters, as they arise in organizations, social institutions and in policy arenas. It would then be necessary to determine who the generational actors are, ascertain what their dominant generational identity might be given the parameters of the situation and examine how this combination influences the value attributed to other generational groups. Mapping would also identify when and where decisions and behaviours take place.

Mapping the generational constituencies would first require identifying which generational groups and positions are tacitly or explicitly involved. This would include those who hold an interest in the outcome and who may or may not be in direct contact with the generational actors in any one context. Second would be to discover or create facilitative spaces for intergenerational communication and decision-making, where the different constituencies can come together in order to negotiate a mutually compatible solution. There is no guarantee that a solution will be found that satisfies all the needs of all parties. However, the possibility of such a space allows voices to be heard in the round and makes it less easy simply to ignore generational issues. The third stage would be to clarify generational priorities. Each party would have the opportunity to critically reflect upon their own generational position, its key features and priorities, establish the degree of overlap with other perspectives and establish similar or complementary roles. Finally, it would be possible to analyse functions and problems with intergenerational insight. By bringing the diverse generational perspectives together, a more complex understanding of the issues emerges, which is likely to lead to sustainable forms of generational collaboration.

Bringing different things to the table

Issues that were once principally uni-generational, in so far as the majority group status was relatively unproblematic and the dominant view obtained by force of numbers, now increasingly appear to be intergenerational. As such, they are in need of negotiation and notions of sustainability themselves would require fresh contact. In an increasingly complex and evenly matched demography, a new settlement is perhaps required. Solutions would need to be seen, not exclusively through the lens of the stewardship of resources from one generation to the next, but also, as numbers of older citizens increase, on ones that build upon multigenerational perspectives in the here and now.

Robert Butler has been reported as saying that gerontology is an amalgam of 'advocacy and science' (Moody, 2001). It has a championing element, as well as a scientific element. It has, historically, championed those who are seen as disadvantaged, downtrodden and rejected by society once their usefulness is done, or as dependent and in need of looking after. The road towards empowerment traced out an ambiguous path between speaking for older adults, and suggesting that 'only older people can talk about old age'. There are good reasons, however, for not allowing any one generation to talk exclusively and unilaterally about itself, just as this is the case in speaking for another generation. Any group is not necessarily the best to articulate a critical perspective on their own condition, or that of their peers. From a generationally intelligent viewpoint, it is important that gerontology moves away from exclusively championing the old and that society moves away from championing youth. A different settlement is needed. The point here is not to advocate negative responses to older people, there are surely enough of these already. But to argue that to fully understand the problems we are facing, we need to critically examine the evasions and eclipses in our own generational positions and their influences on our chosen topic rather than being unself-consciously swept up by them. Until we can work out what it is that each generation brings to the table, what it is about their position in the life-course, family and historical experience that throws a novel perspective on what it is to be human and travelling through time, we will not obtain a genuinely intergenerational solution that can take the measure of the challenges that now face us.

Conclusion

Generational Intelligence constitutes an attempt to move beyond bipolarities of conflict or solidarity and to interrogate intergenerational space. It provides a way of examining the degree to which individuals or groups are capable of seeing from alternative age-perspectives. It also places an emphasis on negotiated solutions and in order to be meaningfully negotiated, this requires an ability to understand the priorities, desires and aspirations of the age-other.

Nevertheless, sustainable intergenerational relationships will need to rely on increased levels of generational insight, empathy and 'intelligence'. Workplaces, care environments, urban and rural spaces and policy decisions are intergenerational, although we tend to see them as age-neutral or with unspoken rules of dominance and priority. We must move beyond the common practice of simultaneously ignoring and acting on the assumption of generational difference.

In this context, Generational Intelligence suggests a framework for understanding contemporary issues and potentially pointing to novel solutions. It prioritizes recognizing difference and commonality, negotiating ambivalence, the discovery of complementary skills and relationships that are mutually recognized, creating facilitative environments in organizations and through social structures. The way in which these tasks might be navigated, is the subject of the rest of this book.

2 Self and the generational imagination

Summary

The purpose of this chapter is to contribute to the development of Generational Intelligence as directed at the self. As such it begins to unpack the first step along the journey towards increased Generational Intelligence, in so far as it addresses the degree to which it is possible to perceive oneself generationally and as distinct from other generational groups. Our everyday encounters with generation are often so subtle and deeply embedded that, paradoxically, we are hardly aware that they are there. Three areas are therefore examined in this chapter that address the way that notions of generation have become a part of the inner world of self. The first includes a look at self-perceptions that are based on age, the second at the emotional figures that inhabit that world and the third, different existential priorities that emerge as the adult life-course progresses. The factors that shape a personal sense of ageing and of generation include images, contents and processes that are generationally constructed. A problem with ignoring these contents and processes is that individuals get stuck in a particular form of generational imagination, which with time increasingly fails to fit their lived experience. A key element for Generational Intelligence then becomes increasing awareness of the way in which people think about their own journey through adult life and how their patterns of thought might change as they move through time and, as a consequence, grow older.

Key points

- Assumptions about age and generation are deeply embedded, but not automatically part of conscious awareness.
- The 'inner world' of the imagination is not age neutral, but includes characteristic ways of thinking about generational content.
- Attitudes to chronological and other forms of age structure self-perception.

- The 'inner life' of the imagination is populated by generational figures that influence emotional responses to others.
- Different phases of the adult life-course hold different existential priorities that can either generate misunderstanding or enrich relationships.

Introduction

The influence of generation and age difference on the way we think and act is often subtle and so deeply embedded that, paradoxically, we are hardly aware that it is there at all. Relationships that are based on assumptions about one's own and different generational characteristics are perhaps most visible in social situations, when one actually encounters people who differ from oneself on the basis of age. Even here, the point at which variation in age becomes a difference in generation is often tacit rather than explicit.

These encounters do not exist in a vacuum, however, and it is important to examine the degree to which habits of thought and even the inner world of the self are structured, as these form foundations for the way responses to age and generation are organized. According to a psychodynamic perspective, for example, everyday encounters constitute the surface manifestations of underlying processes that influence the way that people behave, think and feel about each other. Even at the level of surfaces and impressions, they can constitute a complex dance of half-acknowledged intuitions and associations which, by degrees, make the self and the other known to one another. Unless individuals become conscious of the ways in which their inner world is structured, it is argued, they will act unknowingly and remain the creatures of these deep-seated associations. Contemporary writing on these personal dynamics has primarily focused on gender (Craib, 2001; Elliot, 2002), which is perhaps unsurprising when two key founders of contemporary psychotherapy, Freud (1909/1962) and Jung (1931/1967), both emphasized gender relations as core elements in the formation of adult identity. When viewed through a gerontological lens, it becomes clear that these internal relations also reflect relationships based on age. A mother or father is not simply a powerful and formative influence on the identities of their son's or daughter's sexuality, that power also rests on generational position and these differences can be expected to provoke an important influence on how those children experience age throughout their lives.

It follows that in order to more fully understand attitudes towards personal ageing and generational identities, it is necessary to explore how age shapes our internal imagination. The forms age takes can be expected to influence both personal and social attitudes to related concepts such as generation. Two themes are examined in this chapter. First, we will look at how notions of age and generation are manifested as part of this inner world of self. Second, we will examine how individuals become critically aware of specific age-based identities as the adult life course progresses. The first looks at content and organization, the second at processes that affect the development of a mature identity in midlife and beyond. The key element of Generational Intelligence would concern the way people think about their own journey through adult life and how their patterns of thought might change as they move through time and, as a consequence, grow older. Generation is used in this chapter to describe markers of personal development that arise via changing life-course perspectives, so that at different points in the process of growing older one moves from one generational identity to another. As such, the principal focus of attention is on temporally distinctive phases of adult development, such as early adulthood, midlife and old age, rather than family relationships or socio-historical cohorts. As these are more closely related to age and personal ageing than other generational forms, the terms age and ageing are used in combination with generation, perhaps more so than in other chapters. At root, this chapter concerns processes of maturity, less in the sense of biological change than in the sense of a capacity for critical awareness of the self and an ability to communicate across generational distinctions. Taken together, these elements supply the grounding processes that might affect the construction of the adult self, how this influences the possibility of putting oneself in place of the age-other and the degree to which it is possible to achieve self-understanding in life-course terms.

Contents and awareness of age and generation

There appear to be at least three ways that age and self interact. The first consists of ways in which self-perception is organized. Second, internal images exist in generationally graded configurations, and appear to influence the way the world is thought about. Third, the questions that lend existential meaning to life are often based on age and life-course position.

Internal images of adult ageing

Self-perception and age

A number of studies have shown that when individuals think about their own ageing, they do not do so as if age were a single and homogeneous experience. Rather, personal age is divided into a number of subjective states (Kaufman and Elder, 2002; Bernard et al., 2004; Biggs et al., 2007; Daatland, 2008). In the US, Kaufman and Elder (2002) found that when asked, individuals could easily distinguish between their subjective, social and ideal ages. Discrepancies between these ways of thinking influenced their sense of personal satisfaction. Bernard et al., (2004) used similar distinctions with British respondents, aged in their late sixties and early nineties, in order to assess the effects living in a retirement community, while Biggs et al., (2007) examined perceptions among UK baby-boomers in midlife. In each case, subjective age (or how individuals 'felt inside') and ideal age (how old I would like to be) were generally perceived to be younger than actual (chronological) age and social age (how old others see me); although the majority of respondents said that they were satisfied with their current age. It would appear, then, that respondents understood these ways of dividing self-experience and were familiar with different age-based ways of thinking about the self. They were used relatively easily to interpret personal identity. While awareness of personal ageing was often associated with peripheral physical signs, such as wrinkles and changes to hair colour and thickness among midlifers, these other sources of age-perception were used to negotiate the tension between youthful and maturing selves. Most people had some idea of how old they would like to be and felt themselves to be, even if this did not fit with their actual age or how they thought others might see them. Norlag, the Norwegian database on life-course, Ageing and Generation (Daatland, 2008) has also included questions on how old respondents felt in years and how old they would like to be if they had the choice. Daatland found that discrepancies between the age adults thought they looked, felt and would ideally like to be showed a fairly consistent pattern once they had reached the age of 20, with ideal age becoming progressively younger than the age individuals thought they appeared or felt themselves to be inside. In other words, while people's ideal age may grow marginally older over time, the gap between this, appearance and feeling increased with age.

Researchers have found that these perceptions of age varied in relation to health, wealth and gender. Demakakos *et al.*, (2005) used data from the English Longitudinal Study of Ageing (ELSA), to compare perceptions of actual and 'self perceived' age and found that while perceptions of growing older were not directly affected by wealth, wealthier respondents were more likely to say that midlife ends and old age starts later, regardless of their age or gender. Health status was the most likely factor to influence perceptions of ageing, with poor health acting as an indicator of old age. Daatland (2008) reports that actual age emerged as the main factor against which subjective self-perceptions were compared, with health again being an important influence on subjective age. Degree of self-acceptance, however, was not related to health status, while psychological resources such as a sense of personal agency and high self-esteem tended to add to positive experiences of adult ageing. In another study, Daatland (2008) found that women were less dissatisfied with current age and report negative age changes to start later than men did, which he attributes to women having better coping strategies with respect to age and generational distinction.

Internal generational figures

While psychodynamic approaches to the life course have most commonly been identified with the gendering of identity, they also serve as a useful source of material on age that is rarely captured by other methods. Freud's (1909/1962) observations on an Oedipal crisis, arising at approximately age four, primarily concerns the process of rebellion against and then identification with the same-sex parent. In Freud's work, the resolution of early conflict 'conceptualizes the psyche's entry into received social meanings' (Elliot, 2002: 22) and forms the foundations of social as well as personal capacities for stability and change throughout life. The paths taken in resolving this core crisis continue to influence adult life-course, as each new relationship is encountered. When this approach is critically observed from a gerontological perspective, it is also apparent that identity is maintained through conflict and resolution between actors of different generations (Biggs, 2007) and the resulting formation of adult identity, characterized by Freud (1936) as a civilizing process, also gives a strong indication of who the generational 'bad guys' are. As Larkin's (1971) poem 'This Be The Verse' puts it, parents 'fill you with the faults they had and add some extra just for you'.

The work of the analytic psychologist C. G. Jung (CW: 1939/1967), who first followed then quarrelled with Freud, divided the adult psyche into animus and anima, male and female archetypes that structure identity. While both exist in women and men, one is dominant and the other secondary depending on gender identification. He also identified age-based characters, such as an 'ageless' youth, a heroic adult and a wise elder. These latter figures lend meaning to the priorities and emotional resonances associated with different parts of the life course. Jung is less concerned with conflict than Freud and more concerned with individual pro- cesses of identity formation, he also extended psychological development beyond childhood to include change arising from the adult imagination.

It appears that this imagination is populated with associations and figures that are generationally structured in a number of ways. Counselling psychologists and psychotherapists, for example, have commented on the way that working with older adults reverses the traditional generational dynamic between an older thera- pist and younger client (Knight, 1996; Woolfe and Biggs, 1998; Evans and Garner, 2004). When the client is older, it is possible for emotional associations to arise that reflect a wide spectrum of generational relations beyond that of the conflictual parental therapist and child-patient. In other words, our inner worlds may be orga- nized along lines arising from experience of grandparents and grandchildren, adult relationships between lovers, siblings and contemporaries in addition to those of early development and each of these may appear in intergenerational interaction. The autonomy attributed to such fantasy activity, that it is literally seen to have a life of its own, also has a bearing on the experience of age-based identities within the psyche. Again, it is Jung who elaborates how these might influence the per- ception of the generational other, and in particular the effects of images of older adulthood. Older adults, he argued appear as important archetypal images within the inner world, where archetypes refer to psychological templates that take the form of individual personalities within the imagination. Two key figures, the wise old woman (Weaver, 1973) and man (Middelcoop, 1985) are seen as appearing in dreams, at points of vulnerability and changing life-priorities. Whilst wise elders inevitably reflect cultural stereotypes (Biggs, 1999) and social and historical cir- cumstances (in some of their attributes); their main function in the adult psyche is to act as gatekeepers and guides to an alternative state of being. This arises partly by their reminding presence as persons of a later generation, and partly as a guide to a state of affairs that the active subject has yet to experience. According to this view, negative feelings and resistance towards wise elders reflects their role as harbingers of personal change as much as the properties of old age itself. Indeed, the elder may be perceived differently depending upon the age and life tasks faced by the dreamer (Brooke, 1991).

The point here is that, psychological associations and archetypal figures that become explicit within the detailed scrutiny of the counselling session, also influence everyday thinking, though not necessarily in a conscious manner. Wise elders are potentially transformative images. They may be resisted if they reflect an unwelcome need to move on from the comforting and familiar or be embraced as guides to deeper self-understanding. They are the shadows of future selves.

Existential changes

Growing older requires that individuals live with both an increasing certainty that life is finite and uncertainty as the assumed realities of younger adulthood are questioned. While younger adults might be aware of death, for example, this is usually a distant and unimaginable event such that it is possible to live everyday life as if one were effectively immortal. Personal finitude, however becomes increasingly real as parents die and with the passage of time, the body becomes less responsive and social roles less facilitative. Later in adulthood, contemporaries also die and the body betrays us. Death becomes a certainty that tempers life- planning and attitudes to the personal life course (Biggs, 1999). At the same time, life becomes increasingly uncertain in so far as the youthful goals of personal achievement, physical agency and the assertion of one's will give way to maintain existing levels of personal competence and eventually coping with vulnerability and decline (Baltes *et al.*, 2005). Dittman-Kohli (2005), summarizing findings from the German Ageing Study, found distinctive differences between the responses of younger, midlife and older adults. Responses to the SELE (Self and Life) sentence completion instrument, reflected a shift with age as concerns with social achievement became less central, and existential ones (time, health, death, impermanence, contingency, finitude, etc) more so. Attitudes to the body also shifted, from a preoccupation with sexual and interpersonal attractiveness to physically integrity, competence and fitness. With age, adults become more concerned with what Dittman-Kohli refers to as 'the multiple conservation of personhood' (2005: 283). Dittman-Kohli and Joop (2007) and Samuels *et al.* (1986) argue that as adulthood progresses 'self understanding is required to absorb and redefine changes in the existential and psychological self' (2007: 294).

This self-understanding, and the existential projects associated with it, appears to vary across the adult life course, and have been described with particular experiential clarity by Jung (1932/1967) in his distinction between the first and second halves of adult life. During the 'first half of life', which spans early adulthood up until middle age, personal identity is thought to be consolidated around the personal will which emerges as the constraints of childhood are cast aside. It is enough for the younger adult 'To clear away all the obstacles that hinder expansion and ascent' claims Jung, (CW, 1932/1967. 9: 114) the object of which is to 'win for oneself a place in society and to transform one's nature so that it is more or less fitted in to this kind of existence' (CW, 1967. 9: 771).

The autonomy found in this first half of life is referred to as a considerable achievement, but one which comes at a cost. Jung goes on to say that, while the first half of life feels as if it is a period of increasing freedom from the family of birth, it simultaneously embraces a new element of social conformity, through work and through building new sets of familial relations. As these roles themselves begin to restrict self-development, they give birth to a second existential task. This differs markedly from the persona, or social mask that is created during the first, which is now seen to consist of 'false wrappings' (CW, 1931/1967. 7: 269) and becoming increasingly routine and lacking in vitality. The transition from social conformity to an understanding of deeper levels of personal psychology, Jung calls individuation, and describes it in the gendered language of the time, in the following way:

> A person in the second half of life . . . no longer needs to educate his conscious will, but who, to understand the meaning of his individual life, needs to experience his own inner being. Social usefulness is no longer an aim for him, although he does not deny its desirability . . . Increasingly, too, this activity frees him from morbid dependence, and he thus acquires an inner stability and new trust in himself.
>
> (Jung, 1939/1967, 16: 110)

To cling on to the priorities of the first half of life beyond their existential sell-by date becomes, a form of existential resistance which arises from a failure to adapt to a changing set of life-priorities. Given that most of the subjects of Jung's therapeutic activity were women, it is safe to assume that he is not referring to an exclusively gendered experience and individuation has been described by Samuels *et al.*, (1986) as the process by which persons become themselves, 'whole, indivisible and distinct from others'. A need for social achievement and acceptance during the first half of life, is replaced by a desire for personal coherence and completeness in the second.

Jung's argument suggests that there is some form of pressure, welling up from deeper levels of the self that pushes people towards an expanded individuality as they grow older. Existential transitions in midlife have been observed by Jaques (1965) who associates it with an increased awareness of death, McAdams (1997; 2001) who is concerned with an increased unity of narratives of the self and an ability to create one's own life story and Biggs *et al.*'s (2007) study of accommodation to both youthful and mature identities.

Tornstam (1996), who collected the experiences of Swedish and Danish older adults, indicates that whilst external losses increase in later life, there is an absence of reported loneliness. This ties in with the frequently cited absence of relationship between well-being and disability in later life (Westerhof and Barrett, 2005), where negative changes in physical functioning coexist with increasing self-reported positive well-being. From a younger life-course perspective, this trend appears paradoxical. However, if mediated by a changed perception in existential priorities, a sense of being increasingly at ease with oneself and an ability to absorb the tension between certainty and uncertainty, becomes intelligible. Tornstam (2005) attributes enhanced coping in later life with a process called gerotranscendence:

> The gerotranscendent individual . . . typically experiences a re-definition of the self and of relationships to others and a new understanding of fundamental, existential questions. The individual, becomes, for example, less self-preoccupied and at the same time more selective in the choice of social and other activities.
>
> (Tornstam, 2005: 3)

He suggests that adults approach identity 'more like a Buddhist' as they age which he interprets as an intrinsic drive towards transcendence of the self marked by 'positive solitude' and an increased broad-mindedness. This is complemented by an enhanced awareness of the difference between self and role, in the sense of distinguishing between the development of what is unique about the self rather than conforming to an appropriate social niche and preoccupation with one's job, appearance and ego.

Such processes are connected to more active and complex coping patterns in social situations. Gerotranscendence, and its accompanying attention to existential issues, reflects the development of active coping strategies rather than the defensiveness and social breakdown implied by disengagement from social activity in old age. In other words, increased accommodation to existential threats in later life also generates a qualitative change in attitudes towards life, which are distinctive and adaptive to the point the individual has reached in their own life course.

So, from this brief review of the internal world of ageing, it would appear that the ways that that world is structured is influenced at a number of levels, including different ways of perceiving personal ageing, the imaginative figures that influence emotional responses to others and temporal changes in life-priorities. Self-perception, internal imagery and existential questioning each contribute to the structuring of age relations in the minds of people as they encounter ageing in themselves and age-attributed difference in others.

Generational Intelligence and the organization of the psyche

It has been argued earlier that rather than being neutral territory, the individual imagination is permeated by issues of age and generational identity. With a few notable exceptions, however, these phenomena have been overlooked by practitioners, social scientists and psychologists working on adult development. This would suggest that there is a theoretical and research task at hand to develop intelligence, in the sense of collecting more sophisticated information on the contents and processes associated with both adult ageing and interpersonal perception. This task would include recognition that the often invisible imaginative realities driving intergenerational behaviour and the perception of self require deeper investigation.

The task of becoming generationally aware of the way we experience ourselves and our everyday generational encounters, we would argue, is a necessary first step for increasing Generational Intelligence in daily life, the work of helping professionals and in the creation of policy in this area. In this chapter, three elements that require conscious recognition have been identified, as part of that process. There are most likely more, that as the field develops can be added to the list. The first element reflects the observation that perceptions of self are organized according to the experience of one's own age, not simply as a chronological measure, but as a source of social and emotional location. The perception of one's own age is thereby intimately linked to both the perception of others and also perceptions by others of the ageing self. The second element reflects images that inhabit consciousness or are capable of becoming part of conscious awareness. These images appear to have generational characteristics and be embedded in a wider emotional series of associations with different parts of the life course. They might, therefore, be expected to influence our thought, feelings and behaviour towards age-others. Finally, there appear to be existential elements that give particular phases of the adult life course, distinctive qualities and priorities. These priorities can be expected to shape the relations between self and other and the ways in which personal energy is directed. Differences as well as continuities between generations emerge that arise from changed activities at different points in the life course which may lead to misperception and a failure of understanding between generational groups unless they are exposed and understood. The initial steps towards increasing Generational Intelligence would be to become aware of these influences so that rather than simply acting them out, we can act with them in mind.

3   Developing generational awareness

Summary

In this chapter an examination takes place of the ways in which individuals become critically aware of their personal generational identities. Three elements are examined in greater detail. The first concerns the balance between assimilating external information into existing generational perspectives and accommodating for alternative positions to one's own. The second recognizes the need to separate out from existing relations, which may confuse personal identity with those of significant others, in order to return to them. The act of return allows the distinctiveness of each party to be acknowledged. The third addresses an increasing realization, with age, that it is not enough to be immersed in the priorities of one's own generation and that a more complex reality needs to be engaged with. Each of these elements contributes to the creation of a critical space in which more complex relationships can be tolerated and understood. These elements supply the grounding processes that affect the construction of an adult self, and ultimately the possibility of putting oneself in the place of the age-other. In becoming aware of the ways that that world is structured in the imagination, the ground is cleared for a more nuanced, but less cluttered form of Generational Intelligence.

Key points

- The process of becoming generationally self-aware involves a move away from egocentric thinking and a balancing of assimilation and accommodation towards others based on age.
- The process of increased self-awareness is a core element of increased maturity and Generational Intelligence, which allows people to take their own assumptions into account.
- This can occur through a process of separation, and then return to the age-other, allowing the boundaries between the two to be more clearly seen.
- A shift from a simple state of mind in which one is immersed in a particular generational perspective, to a more complex position, allowing

multiple perspectives to be considered is a marker for increased Generational Intelligence.
- Increased awareness of self and insight into generational others is not only based on differences in age, but also on differences arising from the ageing process itself and relies on recognizing the way our own thoughts and feelings are organized.

Introduction

In the previous chapter, the influence of age and generation was sought in the contents and categories that exist in the individual imagination. If, it was argued, the inner world of self is organized with age in mind, so to speak, then this may be a contributing factor in the apprehension of personal ageing and the recognition of generational difference. Both of these processes would contribute to the development of Generational Intelligence as directed at the self. However, it is, in many everyday situations, possible to 'know something' and behave as if it does not exist, even though the act of denial affects how one behaves. If age and generation are phenomena of this type, if for example, we work as if we are living in a continual present or assume that out attitudes to age are universally valid and unproblematic, it may be that we misread our social environment and even our own futures as well as the circumstances of others. We may assimilate new generational information into existing preconceptions rather than accommodate it in anticipation of deeper understanding.

When on the trail of generational understanding an issue of particular interest would be to see whether there are processes that occur developmentally, that influence the possibility of seeing other people as separate from oneself and, whether these vary by age. In this section, rather than searching for the contents of any one age-relationship and how these determine a person's outlook, emphasis will be placed on the degree to which changes in outlook also lead to changed contents and priorities. As such it picks up on a way of seeing the life course as a more fluid and reflexive process, with a particular emphasis on potential shifts from complacent immersion in the worldview of any one age group, into positions of greater complexity. Under the right circumstances, a critical distance between past and present states of awareness might emerge, that leads to a deeper understanding of the human condition and in particular generational relations.

Different processes have been suggested as ways in which these unthought processes can become known. First, engagement with the imaginative contents identified in the previous section, through an act of 'active imagination', the object of which is to establish a dialogue with internal images associated with the age-other. Second, a process of psychological separation and return, the object of which is to clarify the boundaries between one's own identity in relation to others, based on age and generational position, primarily within families. Third, an existential process which can occur in midlife, is particularly sensitive to the emergence of complex forms of generational consciousness. The process of becoming aware of generational complexity, in other words, appears to be something that takes place in circumstances which are culturally variable and affected by life-course change. Key to each of these is the emergence of a capacity to step beyond a personal assumptive reality and to engage with the other as separate from yet connected to oneself. The process of increased awareness of self and of others becomes a dance in which attention to the movement of one enhances the capacity to respond to the other.

Assimilation, accommodation and adult egocentrism

At every age it appears that people act on the basis of a series of assumptions that explain their perspective on the world, but which at the same time can make it difficult to put themselves in the place of others. For a small child, it may even be difficult to perceive physical events from a different perspective from the one they are in themselves. They assume that everyone sees the same thing from the same position and that that position is the same as their own. This process, called egocentrism, has been defined, in social terms, as an inability to see things from another's point of view (Papalia and Wendkos, 2006). Jean Piaget's (1952) original formulation of egocentrism concerned the cognitive development of children to a point at which they reached adult levels of logical thinking. Once identified, it became clear that these patterns of thought also had a much wider influence on social behaviour and moral judgement (Sugarman, 2000). Judgements about responsibility, the importance of a problem or the perception of feelings were limited by a relative inability to see beyond the boundaries of a particular way of thinking or schema. According to Piaget, these ways of thinking depended on the developmental stage that an individual had reached. An egocentric child was not selfish in the way the phrase is used in everyday speech, rather they failed to see beyond their own particular worldview, which itself reflected their degree of maturity.

Piaget claimed that at any age an egocentric perspective was maintained and changed by two processes. Assimilation allowed new information and events to be included by finding a place for them within the existing schema, while accommodation modified the schema itself in the light of these new experiences. The balance achieved between accommodation and assimilation helped to determine the power of egocentric thinking during any one developmental period. Further research has indicated that forms of egocentrism are by no means restricted to childhood. Adolescence can be marked, for example by a sense that one is living out a unique story that no one else can understand, and, simultaneously that one's every move is subject to collective scrutiny, rather like being continually on stage. Frankenberger (2002) found that notions of a personal fable and an imaginary audience that are used to guide behaviour, forms of egocentrism traditionally associated with adolescence, could be detected as late as in people aged 30 years. In terms of intergenerational perception, Tornstam (2005) has argued that a 'centricity of patterns' of thinking extends into midlife and inhibits an ability to accurately perceive the priorities of old age. He characterizes this form of ego-centrism as 'if everything could just continue unchanged as it is now, life would be at its very best. What lies ahead is nothing to look forward to', which leads to a number of erroneous assumptions about aspects of later life, such as the possibility of fulfilment in retirement and the positive experience of solitude. Biggs (2005) has suggested that at every age, individuals are, in some respects seduced by their own age-specific perspective and that the early midlife values of work-like productivity and social engagement should not be assumed to be the priorities of later years. Both authors have identified midlife as a key period when current preoccupations are projected forward onto later adulthood, creating a mismatch between this age-groups' assumptive realities and the experiences of people who have accomplished the next period of adult development. If adults also experience a form of egocentrism, then it may help to explain certain social phenomena such as Featherstone and Hepworth's (1989) observation that 'midlifestyleism', or the privileging of the priorities of this period of life are pressing ever more deeply into the later years and the finding that baby-boomers actively dissociated them-selves from the characteristics of older age-groups (Biggs *et al.*, 2007). One possible explanation of these behaviours would be a tendency to assimilate alternative perspectives into one's own current preoccupations and a reduced emphasis on the accommodation of alternatives. In contrast to midlifestyles, Tornstam (2005) claims that an important component of the final stage of adult development, is the ability to connect with other generations. While Sadler and Biggs (2006) have, like Tornstam, suggested that a closer affinity to spiritual values characterizes a more naturalistic worldview in later life, even if this is often an anathema to the midlifestyle consumerist project.

Brandtstädter and Rothermund (2002) specifically identify processes of coping with ageing that rely on an optimal balance between assimilation and accommodation. In particular, advancing age is associated with a shift from assimilating new information into existing priorities to an accommodative style that facilitates adaptation to changed circumstances. A third process, immunization, is also described that refers to changing the interpretation of information relevant to the self, most commonly in the service of maintaining a positive self-image. Immunization is seen as a form of self-protection against negative experiences associated with ageing. However, an important distinction between assimilation and immunization is that the former reflects a denial and the latter an avoidance of negative phenomena. Dittman-Kohli and Joop (2007) have linked these processes to adaptive strategies used in old age: selection, optimization and compensation. These strategies, first identified by Baltes and Baltes (1990) reflect ways of coping with restrictions occurring as a person ages while maximizing an individual's autonomy. Selection, for example, refers to concentrating on a more limited number of activities that can be optimized to give the best accommodation to changed circumstances and be used to compensate for other activities that they can then replace. A sports enthusiast may drop a number of high-activity sports, for a more gentle activity, such as Tai Chi, that can then be mastered in order to maintain day-to-day fitness. Age thereby finds accommodation that also maintains elements of personal continuity. Marcoen *et al.* (2007) have suggested that the identification of such strategies broaden an understanding of accommodation and assimilation to include a dynamic of losses as well as one of gains, the negotiation of losses being an increasing factor as older lives progress.

It is interesting to note that these findings suggest that adult ageing brings with it a wider repertoire of accommodative strategies and a dropping of certain forms of adult egocentrism in the later stages of human development. This suggests the opposite to the common belief that individuals grow more rigid and resistant to change with age. Rather than willing new experiences into pre-existing patterns, maturation appears to be closely related to generational intelligent activities, including an ability to modify preconceptions and adapt behaviours whether by choice or by necessity. Thus, according to this approach, generationally intelligent forms of accommodation may occur naturally in some individuals as they grow older. In others, it may be fostered in facilitative contexts or via particular life transitions.

The approaches outlined earlier are primarily concerned with adaptation to everyday events in the immediate present. They describe, in other words, the ways that people deal with information and situations as they rise in front of them and the ways of seeing and thinking that are used to absorb new information or adapt to it. In this sense they touch the surface of generational problem-solving, but do not take account of deeper levels of self-understanding. Individuals are still immersed within the schema they are using and have not become critically aware of it. Little has yet been said about the ways in which influences on intergenerational relations that are not yet recognized, can reach conscious awareness.

Unthought knowns, immersion and reflection

Dittman-Kohli (2005) describes the development of age-identity as a process of 'self understanding and self interpretation, leading to more or less structured self knowledge in the sense of a subjective theory that can function as a cognitive map to orient and motivate behaviour' (2005: 279). In other words, identities not only help us understand who we are at any one point in time, they also give us a sense of direction and reasons for behaving in one way rather than another. This process she sees as a dialogue between certain self-positions: current views of oneself, future aspirations or past roles, which are subject to change across the life course. 'Self-understanding is required to absorb and redefine the changes in the existential and psychological self' (Dittman-Kohli and Joop, 2007). So, for adaptive change to take place, some degree of practical recognition is necessary so that adults can understand their own positions and actively engage with change, rather than simply be swept along by it.

A strange thing about our awareness of difference based on life course and generation is that we all know, at some level that we are ageing and that we make judgements about others based on their age relative to our own. However, in most everyday experiences we simply forget it. Failure to recognize persons on the basis of age and behaviour on that same basis appear to be a commonplace of contemporary life. Working within the psychodynamic tradition, Bollas (1987) has referred to the process of recognition as starting from a position of an 'unthought known'. He is particularly concerned with the effects of childhood experience on adult identity. Here, the unthought known

> Refers to any form of knowledge that as yet is not thought. Genetically based knowledge – what constitutes instinctive knowledge – has not been thought out. Infants also learn rules for being and relating that are conveyed through the mother's logic of care, much of which has not been mentally processed. Children often live in family moods or practices that are beyond comprehension, even if they are partners in the living of such knowledge.
> (Bollas, 1987: 213–14)

In adulthood, these early influences cohere into what Bollas calls an idiom. 'The idiom of a person refers to the unique nucleus of each individual, a figuration of being that is like a kernel that can, under favourable circumstances evolve and articulate'.(Bollas, 1987: 212).

The value of the 'unthought known', to our current inquiry, is that it makes us aware of aspects of the self that are not part of consciousness, but nevertheless are known at some level. Aspects of experience that are suppressed or repressed, for instance, may not currently be part of consciousness. But they had, at one time, to be known in order for their 'forgetting' to take place.

'Unthought knowns' may be particularly helpful in characterizing knowledge, such as our awareness that people age, and the suppression of that knowledge if it threatens our sense of personal identity. The fact that I will age is, in other words, simultaneously known as a condition of human existence and often left unthought as it pertains to ones' personal future. People know that they will age, yet behave as if they are immortal, as if somehow ageing does not apply to them in anything more than at the most superficial level of appearances. This ignoring is perhaps a form of midlife egocentrism. People are carried along in the 'here and now' of working life, for example, rarely paying attention to their pension situation unless an economic crisis forces the issue. Diet and exercise in midlife affect well-being in later life, yet that knowledge is often not used: it has not become part of one's conscious idiom. These examples move beyond Bollas' original meaning that concerns pre-verbal experience in the personal past, and extend the conceptual value of unthought knowledge to the understanding of future events and why, when applied to adult ageing, awareness of personal ageing may be difficult to achieve. As awareness of personal ageing forms the basis of generational awareness, these processes are closely linked.

Bollas concludes that in order 'to facilitate the articulation of the heretofore inarticulate elements of psychic life, or what I term the unthought known. Once the . . . self state is verbally represented, then it can be analysed' (Bollas, 1987: 210). In other words once we are able to speak about generational influences, we can begin to understand them and move beyond their unconscious control. The fantasy of desiring to 'stay young', for example would encounter the mature imaginative process of adapting to changed life-course priorities.

Thus, consideration of the unthought known of adult ageing and inter-generational relations, draws attention to aspects of self-experience that are unconscious but nevertheless stored and influential to generational awareness– the emergence of Generational Intelligence and translation of age difference into social and relational categories. They are suppressed in the service of immediate experience and in this sense known, whilst simultaneously chosen to be ignored in a variety of spheres of life and life-planning. Adults in their thirties may 'know' about old age as an abstraction, but when it comes to thinking about it assume it is in some way 'not me', similarly people in the 'third age' of active retirement may chose not to recognize the 'fourth age' of decline and dependency. That such future states are more often than not subject to negative stereotyping further reinforces their suppression from personal consciousness.

Active imagination, separation to return and maturing imaginations

Given the potential power of the suppression of age-related issues, processes that facilitate an awareness of generational differences come to represent an important factor in adaptation to age-related changes in society. Indeed, when individuals ignore ageing, it does not necessarily reduce their anxiety about their personal futures in terms of their health, wealth or happiness (Biggs, 2008).

'Getting Stuck' and the active imagination

A problem with ignoring the unthought known is that individuals get stuck in a particular form of generational schema, idiom or consciousness, which with time increasingly fails to fit their lived experience. Jung (1961) identified midlife as a time when his patients increasingly felt unable to move forward in life. Similarly, McAdams' (1993) work on narrative counselling indicates that midlife requires an active process of 'selfing' whereby multiple roles, past identities and future directions are built into a coherent life story.

The method suggested by analytic psychology as a means of engaging with unthought parts of the self, has been called 'active imagination' (Chodorow, 1997). For Jung, the great benefit of active imagination was that it enabled individuals to stop being immersed in contents of the imagination, as these appear in dreaming, and other forms of activity that evidence the power of unconscious and imaginal activity such as the elder-archetypes discussed earlier. In dreams, communications from the unconscious are passively received and the dreamer is lost within the world of dreaming. The object of active imagination is to separate out conscious awareness from the imaginative material in order to achieve a dialogue between the two. Dreamers are encouraged to become aware of themselves as an observer of the dream, and by degrees become able to independently engage with the characters that personify certain personal contradictions that are not yet understood.

Chodorow identifies two stages in the development of an active imagination: 'First letting the unconscious come up and second, coming to terms with the unconscious . . . it is a natural sequence that might go on over many years' (1997: 10).

In practice, this first step simply consists of letting things happen, a sort of meditative daydream in which material is allowed to emerge and be consciously observed.

> At first the unconscious takes the lead while the conscious ego serves as a kind of attentive inner witness. Then . . . in the second part of active imagination consciousness takes the lead. As the affects and images of the unconscious flow into awareness, the ego enters actively into the experience. This part might begin with a spontaneous string of insights; the larger task of evaluation and integration remains. Insight must be converted into an ethical obligation – to live it in life.
>
> (Chodorow, 1997: 10)

The difference between active imagination and passive immersion is that previously unthought material can be consciously recognized and properly engaged with and the individual becomes an active player in the narrative as it develops. This is particularly important because our imaginations rely on a series of images of types of people and personalities as templates for generational thinking. The inner world is inhabited in this sense and organized along generational principles. Drawing these images up into conscious levels of awareness permits, over time, a considered recognition of their role in everyday reality and, in so doing, channels their disruptive power. A consideration of the active imagination, as a part of the wider project of making images and associations visible, deepens an understanding of intergenerational processes as they emerge in the internal world of the imagination.

Separation and return

Becoming conscious of one's own generational identity is a force that both links and distinguishes particular generational groups, in so far as it is not until one becomes conscious of one's own distinctive generational idiom that one can develop genuine relationships with other generations. From a psychodynamic perspective, this question translates into the degree to which the 'power' of preceding generations still determines the experience of newly emerging ones. This theme has been taken up by Pincus and Dare (1978) and by Faimberg (2005). Here, the relationship between generations is characterized as one of escape, and mature identity is achieved through a newly found freedom of self-definition, freed from an overbearing influence of preceding generations which has to be recognized to be outgrown. It does not imply a forgetting of the past, rather a new settlement with it. Once the influences of these generations have been identified, it becomes easier to draw a clear boundary between generational selves and others and therefore perceive the other and the self with a newly found clarity.

According to Pincus and Dare (1978), if family cultures subsist on a basis of generational secrets such as unacknowledged deaths, disappearances, rivalries or identities, then 'Secrecy is maintained at great emotional cost, not because it is realistically helpful to anyone, but because everyone is terrified of the assumed consequences of not maintaining it' (1978: 141). These secrets can lead family members to simply re-enact familial preoccupations or unresolved conflicts that may have taken place even before individuals were born and are unconsciously passed on from one generational group to the next. According to this view, adolescence may not simply be a time of experiment and of finding an acceptable fit into an adult identity as 'Teenagers whose behavior indicates their own ambivalence to growing up, can at the same time be expressing any secret ambivalence the parents may have had to their own growing up' (1978: 78). The trick, then, is to discover the generational secret in order to escape its power to repeat patterns across generations.

Faimberg (2005), whose work is based on the notion of 'telescoping of generations', takes this argument further. 'Telescoping' refers to the intrusion of conflicts that existed in preceding generations into the unconscious world of the present generation, whose experiences then becomes 'alienated because they partially depend upon conflicts of a generation that is not the patient's' (2005: 11). The younger generation therefore becomes subject to conflicts and avoidances that they have not directly experienced. She cites as an example, the unexplained loss of relatives during atrocities in the Second World War. These conflicts exist as a paralyzing absence in the current generation who may not even have knowledge of the source of the original events and are at once 'empty and over-full', empty of personal psychological content and stuffed with unresolved material from past generations. According to Faimberg, when stuck in the world of 'telescoping', differences between generations are symbolically collapsed, and there is a sense of time standing still. Once these secrets are recognized, they begin to lose their power and individuals can start to develop their own generational awareness as 'the sense of being outside of the passage of time is overcome' (2005: 12).

Separating out from these unthought materials allows the individual to establish clear boundaries: a space between themselves and the generational other. Once this is achieved, the possibility emerges of being able to 'see' this way of seeing for what it is, and of moving beyond it. It is, in other words, important to escape immersion in a family's unconscious culture in order to see generations clearly. Then the possibility of re-engagement as a separately defined generational being emerges as a precursor to genuine intergenerational communication. The object is to achieve clarity about oneself, clarity about the other as other, and not to confuse the first as an extension of the second.

Becoming conscious of one's own distinctive identity emerges as a force that both links and distinguishes particular generational groups, in so far as it is not until one becomes conscious of generational difference that one can develop genuine relationships between generations.

From simple to complex states of mind

The preoccupation with generational escape in the works of Pincus and Dare (1978) and Faimberg (2005) also draws attention to the experience of being part of a particular generation in adulthood. This is a perspective that Bollas (1992) explores. Rather than taking kinship and the family as his focus, Bollas is perhaps unique in extending psychoanalytic understanding to include cohort difference. 'Sometime in midlife', he tells us 'we become aware of how our generation moves through time' (1992: 263).

The experience of growing older is examined, here, as a differential awareness of self and others that occurs as a result of what he calls 'generational consciousnesses'. This is seen partly as a developmental process through which a more complex sense of self emerges, and partly as a product of changing historical circumstances.

> A generation will have achieved its identity within ten years, roughly speaking between twenty and thirty. In the space between adolescent turbulence and the age of thirty when childhood, adolescence and young adulthood can be viewed of a piece, the thirty year old will feel himself to be part of his generation, and he will, in the next few years, take note of a new generation defining itself in such a way that he can distinguish it from his own.
>
> (Bollas, 1992: 260)

According to this view, the process of becoming conscious of one's own generational position, in a cultural sense, is intimately connected with the emergence of other generational forms. Bollas is no longer talking about awareness of age per se, but age as organized into culturally signified distinctions. With maturity, people cease to be immersed in their own generational culture, become aware that it is no longer the dominant generational form and can increasingly objectify its place in time and as a cultural product. This process clarifies the distinction between becoming aware of one's adult identity, culturally reinforced as an adolescent phenomenon, and a growing awareness of the social distinctiveness of each generational group. As 'A keen sense of their own generation' emerges 'They can define it clearly, differentiate it from older and younger generations, and in some respects analyze why their generation is the way it is' (Bollas, 1992: 252). The older generation is, in this sense, forced into more complex forms of generational consciousness as its 'precious objects are discarded on the heap of history'.

It appears then that the generational consciousness of midlife is distinguished from the emerging will of young adulthood. It is more melancholic, rueful and pained as its achievements are passed by. The task of generational consciousness is no longer a process of removing the unwanted baggage of preceding generations. The mantle of novelty, youthfulness and of carrying a collective hope for the future is replaced by a growing recognition of the contingency of one's own personal relationship to social and historical development. It now requires a considered distinction between mature adulthood and the immediacy of youthful experience.

No longer escaping the power of preceding generations, the mature adult has to come to terms with the emergence of new generations and the personal passage of social time.

The relationship between the newly emerging and the preceding generation is an interesting one in so far as it adds further insight into the nature of youthful adult egocentrism. The emerging generation must know of the existence of other generations, while simultaneously discounting them. It is engaged in a process of self-definition, rather than relational definition. The process of coming to terms with generational complexity is left to the older generational group. As Bollas puts it, and forgiving his rather arcane insensitivity to gendered speech:

> Each new generation is a period of intense subjective life, a time for the simple self who feels himself to be part of a collective process carrying him along inside it. Music, fashion, lingual expressions, social idioms, seems to give immediate expression to the parts of the self which take their place in the plenitude of generational objects. This period on the immersion of self in the culture gives way in and through time to the complex self who collects these selves into one more or less objectifiable location when one reflects on those selves as objects. In the course of generational progression one is less immersed in social culture, less idiosyncratic and more conventional, and increasingly inclined to see the self and its objects more clearly. This is in part what is meant by wisdom; that knowledge accrued out of reflected upon experiences.
>
> (Bollas, 1992: 270)

The complexity that is born out of new boundaries being set between the midlife and the emerging generation contributes here to a reflective objectication. One becomes distanced from oneself, and in so doing allows a certain critical distance and control over intergenerational activity. Simple self-states, as dominated by the adult will, are caught up in immediate experience, instinct and feeling. They are rather like Berger and Luckman's (1966) depiction of 'commonsense reality' whereby socially structured events and attitudes are accepted at face value. They are assumed to be the only credible reality, rather one of a number of inter-subjectively created possibilities. They are held in common and rarely reflected upon. Although one cannot help thinking that as emerging generations often define themselves in contra-distinction to the world they find before them, that the ego-centrism of emerging generations is to recognize but simultaneously discount their impact on existing generational groups. In a complex state, one observes oneself as an object 'from the outside' allowing 'deep experiencing' to take place. According to Bollas, then, the first experience of generational belonging, as new generations emerge, carries its members along in an unreflective collective process – a time for the simple self. In the course of generational progression, individuals become less immersed in their own generational culture, and increasingly inclined to see the self and others as socially contingent. The ultimate consequence of this process is a more complex and nuanced relation to generational identity.

It appears, that the emerging recognition of generational interdependence is accompanied by a growing facility for complex states of mind. Simple immersive states give way to complex reflective ones. The first is a captive of its own terms of reference, and the second draws on a mixture of accumulated experience, changing social priorities and maturation through the life course to put its own identity in context. Bollas draws an analogy, here, between dreaming and self-awareness: 'similar to progression from the world of sleep and dream, when one is a simple self inside the process, to the awakened and conscious complex self who reflects upon the experiences as an object'. (Bollas, 1992: 270).

Each of the processes described previously identify the need for distance between the immediate surfaces of experience and deeper levels of reflective awareness. In ceasing to be immersed, a distinction is achieved between different aspects of generational identity that allows critical reflection to take place. At each level; in using active imagination to distinguish between conscious and unconscious activity; separating and returning to the self in the realm of the family; and, in examining developing awareness of cultural differences between generations, Generational Intelligence-like processes are intimately related to the recognition and redefinition of personal boundaries. In order to achieve intergenerational understanding, boundaries must be both clearly identified while allowing certain permeability so that genuine communication, between levels of self-awareness, as a basis for communication between self and others, can be achieved.

From generational awareness to Generational Intelligence

The primary focus of this and the preceding chapter has been the degree to which a conscious awareness of generation takes place and how that is affected by different levels of psychological activity. As such a spotlight has been trained on how Generational Intelligence can be applied to the self, the balance achieved between assimilation of and accommodation to other influences and the transition from simple to more complex states of mind. Self-awareness thereby becomes the initial step towards greater generational insight and a clearing away of barriers and self-deceptions that would inhibit intergenerational understanding.

In terms of Generational Intelligence, awareness of inhabiting a generational position does seem to vary depending upon how far one has progressed through the adult life course, especially in terms of capacity to recognize alternatives. This has been described as a shift from immersion to one of critical distance, and from assimilation to accommodation. While many aspects of adult ageing are left out of everyday thinking, we all know that, we are likely, if we are lucky, to grow old and have some memory of what it was like to inhabit earlier periods of life. In contemporary society, most of us put this in brackets together with the associations and internal figures that influence emotions and attitudes towards age-others. In terms of the argument pursued in this book, concern lies with the relative ability to engage with alternative positions, because this opens the way to understanding personal existential priorities and in cognizance of the position of others. As has emerged, as identified in the preceding chapter, the 'others' one is talking about also inhabit the internal world of the individual rather than simply existing as separate individuals in the outside world. Problems arise when those 'real' others are seen through the lens of these internal images and assumptive structures. It is part of the job on Generational Intelligence to see these assumptive realities for what they are and not to confuse them with actual members of other generations. So, to see the other more clearly, to put oneself in their place, the influence of the internal image has to be understood. Separation from and return to the other, both internally and externally, is necessary in order to act with an awareness of ones' own generational circumstances. Failure to do so would lead to an assumption that other positions hold the same priorities as ones' own and thus eclipse other generations as consisting of separate beings, a form of generational egocentrism.

Similarly, to act with an intelligence of one's personal generational circumstances means to be clear that one is responding to the priorities of the part of the life course one is in, rather than adopting them from another generational position. Not to do so can lead to mistaking one set of generational priorities for another, and can often happen if a different point in the life course is afforded greater status, or the position held is negatively valued. The temptation is then to deny or avoid attributes authentically relevant to the self, which are not given social value. The point, pursued in this chapter, is that the potential to understand the way that life course positions embed and are embedded in our inner worlds, promises the freedom to act with what one could think of as generational freedom. This, however, is less a form of generational trimphalism, as a capacity to transcend particular generational constructions. In such circumstances, one gets an inkling of how to act in accordance with generationally intelligent priorities. Such a shift would have to make sense in terms of the intrinsic processes of adult ageing, while simultaneously taking into account the alternative generational arrangements of others. So-to-act means to act authentically relative to the rhythms of the life course and how far one has travelled down its pathways.

4 Self and other

Summary

In turning to the relationship between self and other, this chapter introduces the problem of empathy between generations. This has been conceived as the relative ability to put oneself in the place of the generational other, and as such would be a key element in developing high levels of Generational Intelligence. A significant roadblock to the development of such empathy, would be forms of social ageism, which can take the shape of the imposition of a dominant age-group's priorities onto other groups whose own life-priorities are then eclipsed. The recognition that the age-other is in some way different, also creates a problem of how to work with people of different age groups and generations. Generational consciousness has often been conceived as the awakening of a sense of generational identity in one group, which can lead to conflict between it and other groups. This can be contrasted with a state of generational solidarity. It is suggested that rather than taking one end of this opposition, between conflict or solidarity, a generationally intelligent approach would attempt to make sense of both, allowing a relative ability to act with awareness of one's own generational circumstances, while also taking the priorities of other groups into account.

Key points

- Generational identities exist in the space between one person and another who are recognized as being of different age groups.
- Recognizing the 'age other' in such a way raises the question of how to understand similarities and differences.
- Making a bridge to the age-other requires degrees of generational empathy.
- Negative social attitudes and practices, such as ageism, create a barrier to empathy by placing the priorities of the dominant generation onto others.
- Dominant discourses include assumptions of conflict and of solidarity which divide intergenerational relations into binary opposites.

Introduction

The otherness of other people raises questions about how they can be understood. And this in turn depends upon the dominant ways in which identities are made available and legitimized by wider social forces. As Dannefer (2008) points out 'everyday social relations are the invisible and unnoticed water we swim' (2008: 6). And part of the move towards generationally intelligent relations would be to make these invisible or taken-for-granted assumptions about the age-other visible. This, he calls the 'missing middle' between personal assumed realities and macro-social phenomena. The surrounding environment, the discourses that shape people's understanding of themselves and others in social space, are key to the relative capacity to place oneself in the position of the age-other and thereby, understand their thoughts, feelings and actions.

One of the main lessons of the previous chapter on generational awareness has been that what at first examination appears to be a closed, internal world of thoughts and feelings about adult ageing, is in fact highly permeable. Internal formations of the age-other are widespread, as are different self-perceptions based on competing conceptions of personal ageing. These often arise from an interaction between personal experience and internalized, socially sanctioned, images of the relationships between age, oneself and other generational groups. If that chapter was primarily concerned with looking inside, we make an attempt, in this chapter, to look outside and link the inner world of self with the dominant ways of seeing others, based on age and generation.

Our starting point, then, is to pose the question: 'how far is it possible to place oneself in the shoes of another adult, when that person is designated as being of a different age-group?' This task seems, on first inspection, to be a relatively easy thing to do. We are all human and we and our neighbours appear to have much in common. However, the closer one looks at the issue, the clearer it becomes that it is extraordinarily difficult to disentangle personal associations and beliefs from what another person might actually be thinking or feeling. These difficulties are enhanced because we are concerned with adult ageing, which is at once poorly defined and subject to negative social attitudes. Social ageism exaggerates negative differences between younger adulthood, midlife and old age. It privileges the priorities of dominant age-groups and their conceptions of what it might be like to be at different points in the life course. If it is accepted that such a social environment is commonplace, the possibility of identifying 'false-positives', things that one believes to be true, but are in fact misconceptions, is also relatively strong.

Here, our discussion of Generational Intelligence centres on three elements of this process. First, the relative capacity to put oneself in that place – to empathize with another person. This does not, as an encyclopedia entry on Empathy tells us, necessarily imply compassion, sympathy or concern (Wikipedia, Empathy, 23/6/09: 1). It does, however address the processes involved in recognizing the separate, yet related position of another person and the ways in which that distance can be filled, positively and negatively. Second, the relationship between personal and structural meaning systems. This has been the particular concern of thinkers in the critical psycho-social tradition, especially with respect to the ways in which social policy influences interpersonal relations within helping systems. Here it is used to analyse the concept of social ageism in more detail. Third, public discourses on intergenerational relations are, more often than not, posed in terms of conflict or solidarity. These opposite poles of attraction, surface manifestations of an underlying debate on what is meant by legitimate social conduct, are critically placed in the same and therefore ambivalent, space.

Empathy and roadblocks to it

Bauman, in his book *Liquid Love* (2003), argues that:

> in contemporary social interaction, individuals are so desperate to relate; yet wary of the state of 'being related' and particularly of being related 'for good', not to mention forever, since they fear that such a state may bring burdens and cause strains they neither feel able nor are willing to bear, and so may severely limit the freedom they need – yes, your guess is right – to relate.
>
> (Bauman, 2003: viii)

His point, for current purposes, is that while we wish to create a bridge to other people, we are severely limited in our capacity to do so by a tendency to focus on the satisfactions any relationship is expected to bring. We exist, in our inevitably social sea, attempting to chart a course between what he calls 'the pleasures of togetherness and the horrors of enclosure' (Bauman, 2003: xi). He follows Heidegger in believing, however, that the frustration that such contradictions cause, lead to an increased level of consciousness about the relationships themselves.

This observation chimes well with Elliot (2002), who claims that the current focus of psychoanalysis is 'not one of individuals suffering from disturbances in sexual repression and self control, but rather that of individuals experiencing a deep emotional poverty in relations with others' (2002: 26).

Within the psychodynamic framework, the resolution of generational conflict holds a key role in 'civilizing' human beings, making them capable of social identification, love and being able to see things from another's perspective. It 'conceptualizes the psyche's entry into received social meanings' (Elliot, 2002: 22) and forms the foundations of social as well as personal capacities for both stability and development. This can be seen in the resolution of Oedipal conflict, in which the child at first wishes to destroy and then, deterred by the perceived retaliatory threat, comes to identify with his or her same-sex parent, the echo of which is heard throughout the life course as each new relationship is encountered. While psychoanalysis has primarily been evoked to understand the formation of gender identity, and it is unclear how far the Oedipal relationship is historically determined, it has, nevertheless, had a profound influence on the cultural understanding of generational relations for most of the twentieth century. An example, specifically addressing relations between adult children and their ageing parents, can be found in De Beauvoir's (1970) *La Vieillesse*, published in English as 'Old Age'. 'The characteristic mark of the adult's attitude toward the old', she tells us,

> Is its duplicity. Up to a certain point the adult bows to the official ethic of respect for the aged . . . But it is in the adult's interest to treat the aged man as an inferior being and to convince him of his decline.
>
> (De Beauvoir, 1970: 245)

Thus adult children are seen to manipulate their ageing parents in order to supplant and ultimately destroy them in an act of delayed Oedipal revenge. As De Beauvoir goes on to say, the older generation becomes a 'different species', one in which it is difficult to recognize oneself, making their elimination easier to contemplate.

An antidote to this state of affairs, balanced finely between interpersonal insecurity, rivalry and conflict with the age-other, is the possibility of empathy. Berger (1987) describes empathy as 'the capacity to know emotionally what another is experiencing from within the frame of reference of that other person, the capacity to sample the feelings of another or to put oneself in another's shoes' (1987: 7). It has most famously been espoused by the psychologist, Carl Rogers (1959), as an ability 'to perceive the internal frame of reference of another with accuracy and with the emotional components and meanings which pertain thereto as if one were the person, but without ever losing the "as-if" condition'.

Empathy, then, includes feeling as well as thinking about the other, recognizing that frames of reference will differ and cannot be assumed to be the same. It implies that there is a way in which it is possible to 'sample' perspectives that are driven by differences of gender, culture and age. That the age-other, in other words, is not a closed book, different species or foreign country.

Engaging in empathic interaction involves a combination of observation, memory, knowledge and reasoning, to generate complex forms of psychological inference (Ickes, 1997), and can be recognized in others when the significance of one's own values and motivations are somehow acknowledged in a way that can be tolerated (Schwartz, 2002). Since it concerns the understanding of positions held by others, the way it evolves is closely related to existing meaning domains others inhabit and the forms of interaction that arise from them, which may be permissive or disruptive of interpersonal insight.

Generational Intelligence poses the question – under what social conditions is fellow-feeling with the age-other possible and how do differences in power and perspective replace one age-perspective with another. And here, it is taken to mean the ability to tune into the thoughts and feelings of groups classified as others, without becoming confused as to the boundaries between self and other, and being mindful of the socially constructed discourses that influence what is recognized.

The relationship between the personal and the social

Key to understanding intergenerational relations, then, is an examination of the relationship between the personal and the social. We need 'a politics which attends to the subjective and emotional experiences . . . alongside issues of redistribution and social justice' (Stenner and Taylor, 2008: 416). Stenner and Taylor argue that the psychological and social elements of relationships have been 'thought separately' and that 'the social life of the psychic world and the psychic life of social forms' (2008: 433) need to be seen, not only as distinct expressions of a process that is unified in experience, but also as one that is deeply enmeshed in wider questions of power. Their main concern is the role of social welfare as a means of inclusion into society which also regulates and administers 'a vast swathe of disadvantaged people', which Phillipson has pointed out (1998) has been the principal means of locating older adults in a wider social context. And, by Grenier (2007) as a means of publicly managing the subjective experience of later life, either as a threat or as an actuality.

Once these experientially unified, yet conceptually distinct elements are brought together again, visibly, and in a space that facilitates critical comparison, it becomes clear that fantasy and reality are closely related. It becomes, as Frosh puts it, that 'Fantasy is not "just" something that occupies an internal space as a kind of mediation of reality, but that it also has material effects, directing the activities of people and investing the social world with meaning' (2003: 1554). Fantasy, then fuels politics and is constantly in tension between inner and outer worlds, self and other, the personal and the public. Frosh argues that 'Just as we need a theory of how "otherness" enters what is usually taken as the "self", so we need concepts which will address the ways in which what is "subjective" is also found out there.' (p. 1555).

As has been shown in the preceding chapter, when analysing the processes that contribute to the self-awareness of adult ageing, internal and external images of ageing and generation are closely connected. The process of placing oneself in the shoes of the age-other, as a preliminary step towards critical intergenerational engagement, also implies a way of questioning the processes that place the 'age-other' as 'not me' and as something to be avoided and denied, particularly when positioned as an older generation.

Ageism

If the possibility of empathy between generations suggests a bridge towards greater intergenerational understanding, then social ageism presents a significant barrier. It is the troll that waits to jump out and scare the younger generation away from encounters with the wider world of generational complexity.

One of the earliest, and most commonly cited definitions of ageism, comes from Butler (1987):

> Ageism can be seen as a process of systematic stereotyping of and discrimination against people because they are old, just as racism and sexism accomplish

this for skin colour and gender . . . Ageism allows the younger generations to see older people as different from themselves, thus they subtly cease to identify with their elders as human beings.

(Butler, 1987: 22)

Here, ageism is placed in the context of wider civil rights issues, as a matter of discrimination and prejudice. The process by which it works is an intergenerational 'othering', which allows dominant generations not to identify with older adults. As the concept has been developed, it grew an institutional dimension as:

A set of beliefs originating in the biological variation between people and relating to the ageing process. It is in the actions of corporate bodies, what is said and done by their representatives, and the resulting views that are held by ordinary ageing people, that ageism is made manifest.

(Bytheway, 1994: 14)

Bytheway places emphasis on both the role of organizations and the way in which their positions are internalized by the objects of their activity. Levi and Banaji (2002) note that it constitutes 'An alteration in feeling, belief or behaviour in response to an individual's or group's perceived chronological age' which is thought to be implicit in everyday situations and influences the outcomes of interaction. The process involved has been elaborated by Biggs (2004) as a form of age-imperialism: 'The colonization of the goals, aims, priorities and agendas of one age-group by another. This may be consciously done for reasons of political and economic expediency, or unknowingly as if these priorities are simply commonsense' (2004: 103).

According to this last definition, one that explicitly engages with the relationship between the personal and the social, ageism occurs consciously or unconsciously. Members of a dominant age-group or generation unthinkingly assume that their perceptions are universally valid. It becomes an unthought known of the intergenerational encounter, where age dominance takes superiority for granted in such a way that its accompanying reality replaces or overrides alternative positions. A result is an unwillingness to consider difference based on adult age, except when that serves the dominant group's interests and in which the dominant view acquires a moral dimension. As Phillips *et al.* (2010) point out,

Every individual has the potential to experience discrimination or prejudice based on their age if they live long enough. It produces an 'othering' effect that lumps all those considered old into a category defined, first, as different and, secondly as inferior. More importantly, it suggests that all old people are alike, hence obscuring differences that exist among and between older persons.

(Phillips *et al.*, 2010: 21)

These authors report a pervasive yet 'uncritically analysed force', with 77 per cent of older adults experiencing verbal ageism, but little outright discrimination.

Coupland (2004) claims that this form of communication is sanctioned by the use of productivity as a criterion for social worth, which becomes the boundary between those at the core and periphery of society. Where older adults are no longer seen as being productive, they become 'aged aliens'. In deep old age, Hazan (2011) maintains that existential priorities become so different from younger age-groups that a form of autism governs attempts at intergenerational communication, and this absence of meaningful interaction renders the old-old disposable.

O'Hanlon and Coleman report that the recipients of negative attitudes are less motivated, more anxious and less able to interact with intergenerational others. Further, a negative attitude to one's own ageing was found to be the best predictor of low self-esteem in later life. Citing a study taking place over 13 years, they note: 'Such evaluations are likely to develop over many decades and become inevitably intertwined and indistinguishable from what we ordinarily think of as development and ageing' (2004: 32).

The reasons why older adults are subject to these attitudes have been subject to multiple interpretation. Martens *et al.* (2005) argue that elders are 'othered' as a psychological defence against fear of death and frailty. Donlon *et al.* (2005) report that frequency of TV viewing is correlated with ageism, while Hepworth (2004) points to the cult of youth in popular culture and Robinson *et al.* (2007) have cited the negative portrayal of older characters in children's entertainment, for example in Disney films. Hagestad and Uhlenberg (2005) and Kohli (2005) both emphasize the role of institutional age-segregation, such as in schooling, health care and in residential homes, which reduces contact between generational groups. It is perhaps unsurprising, then, that Help the Aged, when undertaking a campaign on the future of health care, claimed:

> Ageism and ageist assumptions run through our services and society. They affect legislation, policy and practice and the attitudes that older people encounter day by day. Pervasive ageism erodes self esteem and undervalues the roles older people play in the lives of their families and communities . . . and deprives the rest of society of the benefits its older members could bring. It needs to be challenged wherever it is found.
>
> (Help the Aged, 2000: 5)

This was shortly followed by a statement in the National Health Service (NHS) National Service Framework for Older People (2001, reviewed 2005) that: 'NHS Services will be provided, regardless of age, on the basis of clinical need alone. Social care services will not use age in their eligibility criteria or policies, to restrict access to available services' (2001: 7).

Negative social attitudes towards older adults has been cited as a permissive element in extreme social phenomena such as elder abuse (Phillipson and Biggs, 2001) and in the cases of serial-killing such as in the Shipman case (Gilleard, 2008) and other examples of age-based murder by nursing staff as reported in Austria (2004), the UK (2008) and Finland (2010).

If it is accepted, as writers as diverse as Dittman-Kohli (2005) and Jung (1931) have maintained that people, in what have been called the first and second halves of adult life, have markedly different life-priorities. Then the imposition of the goals, aims, priorities and agendas of one age-group onto and into the lives of other age-groups forms a considerable barrier and a target for intergenerational empathy. If generationally dominant priorities are simply thought of as common sense, especially when one happens to be in the dominant age-position, then an unwillingness to consider diversity based on adult age allows the most power-ful perspective to acquire a moral dimension. If one ends up on the wrong side of this equation, one lives one's life according to principles that are out of kilter with emerging life-priorities, and in some cases, circumstances that give licence to motivations seeking to eliminate, symbolically and in extreme cases, corporally, the older generation.

Following Bauman, age imperialism would form a case specific example of a wider social trend towards human disposability. In a statement that prefigures Hazan's (2011) analysis of the very old, Bauman critiques contemporary social val-ues as exemplified by a catalogue of game-shows in which contestants team up to defeat weaker participants, in the service of longer term self-interest, as eventually each has to compete with another. 'These TV spectacles that took millions of view-ers by storm and immediately captured their imagination were public rehearsals of the *disposability* of humans' (Bauman, 2004: 88) The root metaphor for these forms of entertainment, he argues are the values of the concentration camp. And who is more disposable, less valuable, less productive and therefore less worthy of public love, than the old? Why invest in someone who will not be around long enough to provide a return on one's emotional and social investment?

The tacit deletion of older generations, the expunging of agency and replace-ment by their active age-other can be found in some unlikely places. So often referred to as 'dignity' in discourses on age and most often conceived in terms such as 'dignity on the ward', is on close inspection a quality afforded to older people by the conduct of others. Dignity in this sense is the gift of the active other and its visibility is contingent upon relations of power and dependency. Another form of dignity, expressed through self-worth, 'character' and 'resilience' by the older person themselves, is less often addressed. The latter emphasises an active role for older adults who may, through their own agency, take responsibility for who they are. The dominant interpretation of dignity, paradoxically reflects the agency of the active and potent who can be carried along in a generational 'time for the simple self'. One is easily immersed in its moral certitude, it does not read-ily throw up issues that make you have to stop and think. On stepping out of that immersive space, however, the question of a personal generational identity and intergenerational dignity become problematic.

Generational consciousness

In addressing the process of Generational Intelligence through the lens of empathic understanding and its opposite in social ageism, our argument stands in an iterative relationship to at least two existing traditions. First, is a tradition assuming conflict, which is dominant in psychodynamic thinking and in European sociology (Biggs, 2007). The second arises primarily from the North American study of the family which starts from an assumption of solidarity between generations (Lowenstein, 2007). And while the two concepts interact, for example in Bengtson *et al.*'s (2002) attempts to include conflict within a solidarity framework, and in European social policy emphasizing 'solidarity between generations' (Johansson *et al.*, 2007), they have been characterized as opposites. Both, however, throw a particular light upon intergenerational relations, and as such represent dominant discourses on the motivations driving generational exchanges.

Within the European tradition, Karl Mannheim (1928/1952) began a sociological discussion of how a generational cohort that at first simply has common characteristics, develops into a self-conscious group with a shared identity. In his essay 'The Problem of Generations', he outlined the key elements in what has come to be called 'Generational Consciousness' (Pilcher, 1994; Edmunds and Turner, 2002; 2005; Gilleard and Higgs, 2005). The principal focus of this work has been an analysis of the role of generations in social change, which was thought to occur through social and historical circumstances that make the emergence of collective experiences more likely to arise. Individuals or groups can, through becoming part of a particular 'generational style', develop a conscious identity based on their shared generational location. Sharing a generational location, such as being born at approximately the same time, holds the potential of becoming, in Mannheim's words, a 'generational actuality' whereby a group recognizes itself as having a shared identity and common interests when compared to other generations. The move from location to actuality, which has since been interpreted as resembling the way in which a social class moves from being simply 'in itself' to one that acts collectively 'for itself' (Turner, 1998), shifts social actors from holding certain experiences in common, to developing a politicized generational consciousness. While this formulation links periods of accelerated social change and generational identity, Mannheim also claims that the advent of any new generation gives the opportunity for 'fresh contact' with a culture's accumulated heritage, and a chance for reappraisal. New generations are therefore seen as an important means of ensuring social renewal and adaptation to changing conditions as it 'teaches us both to forget that which is no longer useful and to covet that which has yet to be won' (Mannheim, 1952: 294).

The development of new generational styles, Mannheim claimed, gave individuals 'a common location in the social and historical process' it also 'limit(s) them to a specific range of potential experience, predisposing them for a certain characteristic type of historically relevant action' (1952: 291).

Both the traditions of psychoanalysis and generational consciousness positions agree that the first step towards personal awareness and social consciousness is the recognition that one is part of a generation. While psychoanalysis places this in childhood with the resolution of the Oedipal rivalry, Mannheim saw the point of reaching adolescence or young adulthood as a time of particular sensitivity to wider social and historical change. Also, if a particularly forceful and iconic generation emerges, this will influence the identities of subsequent generations as it forms a reference point that both highlights the role of that generation and the salience of 'generation' as a social and historical category. One is part of, or lives in the shadow of, the generation that acted out its common destiny.

So, individuals have variable access to generational consciousness depending upon their historical experience. Some generations are therefore more real than others in cultural terms, as is the degree to which social change is expressed in terms of generational tension. Mannheim gave the example of political youth groups in early twentieth century Germany. A more recent example might be the '60's generation, in western culture, or the Global IT generation of the 1990s (Edmunds and Turner, 2005). In each case social change occurred in harness with a culturally recognized step-change in generational relations.

Generational style has also been used to emphasize the way that certain cultural habits and preferences act as a focus for consciousness and identity. Corsten (1999), for example, explores the concept of the 'cultural circle' as formative of generational consciousness. Rather than simply being products of historical events, generational identities are seen as something sustained by interpersonal interaction. Generations, it is argued, consist of 'people who spontaneously observe that other people use certain criteria for interpreting and articulating topics in a similar manner to themselves' (p. 262). Some authors, have attempted to fuse 'generational style' with Bordieu's concept of 'habitus' (Edmunds and Turner, 2005; Gilleard and Higgs, 2005), and point to specific lifestyles that sustain and reinforce 'within-generation' consciousness. Generational groups and individuals can live within their own particular habitus, which creates a more flexible generational space than historical context alone. However, this emphasis on creating a particular lifestyle 'bubble', does not say very much about inter-generational relations, other than in the ability to recognize similar or dissimilar habitus-dwellers. It is, paradoxically, given its strongly social credentials, about the formation of identity within a generation rather than empathic exchange between generations.

Generational consciousness and conflict

It would come as no surprise then, that emerging generational consciousness has been associated with intergenerational conflict. Turner (1998) has identified the notion of generational conflicts as 'a structural aspect of social struggles over limited resources' (1998: 299). He makes the case for significant and growing generational conflict based on cohort difference, and expressed in terms of lifestyle and economic power. So 'positive opinions towards elderly individuals, which may be structured by norms of either reciprocity or beneficence, can coincide with a considerable degree of generational hostility and conflict over scarce resources' (1998: 301). Events such as the 'sixties generation' are seen as an attempt to rebalance inequalities, which at the time took the form of a younger generation experiencing social changes in gender relations, cosmopolitanism and multiculturalism. As that large cohort moves through time, however, it itself comes to engage in practices that exclude newly-emerging generations through emphasizing its own commonly held habits, popular culture and taste. These practices are intended to prevent succeeding generations from accessing the resources held by the dominant generational group through 'credentialism' and by privileging 'generationally marked experiences'. In casting generational rivalry in terms of blocking the rise of new generations, Turner reverses the position in which the younger generation drives any conflict. However, rather than bleaching out a radical interpretation of generational impact, Turner highlights its effect on personal age-consciousness and in creating 'in' and 'out' groups to maintain public forms of generational power. At root, the 'problem' of the sixties generation, from Turner's perspective is still a problem of succession. They are, in later life, seen as excluding the rise of the next generation through an overbearing sense of their own, yet outmoded, generational identity. Edmunds and Turner (2005) continue to stress the role of antagonistic social relations and processes in the formation of generational consciousness. They argue that, in the twenty-first century, this process has become global in nature, so that 'globally experienced traumatic events may facilitate the development of global generations' (p. 564). Such generations are defined as being similar to the 'sixties' or baby-boomer generation, who forged strong generational symbols and emotive connections through youth-driven social movements and the consumption of goods and services. Twenty-first century generations are, however, facilitated through developments in communications technology, or an international crisis such as 9/11. They further note that technology is now salient in the formation of generational consciousness but they argue that such global generations are not homogeneous and vary according to national, regional and local differences in technological access and in the interpretation of events.

To some extent, these forms of intergenerational dissatisfaction reflect the 'progress' narratives to be found in twentieth century modernism, where generational consciousness has, in common with psychoanalysis, a tendency to cast the older generation as a brake on social progress. They accentuate the urgency of novel solutions to intergenerational questions and that in the current period, social conflict has the potential to be expressed in generational rather than other terms. A shrunken demographic middle, created as economically productive age groups stay in education for longer, retire earlier and live for longer (see, for example, the EC Lisbon Agenda), may have contributed to this sense of scarcity and competition. It has certainly become associated with the so called 'boomer' cohort as this relatively large demographic group reach the traditional retirement age (Biggs *et al.*, 2006). It may also reflect attributions of responsibility and stewardship with respect to environmental issues (Dobson, 2000). Trends in pensions policy, to give but one example, may be expected to exacerbate intergenerational rivalry. Driven by wider economic concerns, and unwillingness to balance lifetime social contributions to current macroeconomic interests, such policies, that expect the younger generation to pay for the older, simultaneously exclude them from the same benefits in their own old age. An exit by employers from established pension contributions (Turner, 2002) exacerbates these effects. Such policies break the contract between citizen and state and employee and employer in ways that are generationally inspired. A spiral of generational disenfranchisement can occur as attempts to reduce current pension entitlements are also used to reduce the entitlement of future generations. Both ecologically and economically, the mess we are in and the burdens of history are issues that are increasingly generationally inflected.

Generational consciousness and Generational Intelligence

If the Mannheimian tradition answers the question of how one becomes conscious of being part of a generation primarily in terms of external social and historical circumstances, and psychoanalysis, in terms of rivalry in early childhood, then Generational Intelligence refers to their interaction, as a process linking changing social experience with personal intellectual maturation and familial circumstance. Each would contribute to a personal sense of generational identity, although the salience of cohort, family or life course position in everyday experience, as being the primary domain of intergenerational relations, would vary depending upon cultural and historical circumstances.

The main distinction between generational consciousness and Generational Intelligence is that whereas generational consciousness privileges the experience of a single generation, Generational Intelligence attempts to bridge generational differences through empathic understanding. In this sense, generational consciousness is immersive, in so far as it is primarily concerned with the rising self-awareness of one, often younger, generational group. It recognizes difference, but principally as a foil to the emergence of a younger group's identity and in the service of overcoming opposition to its own ascendancy. It is not immersive simply in the sense of not recognizing the age-other as having a distinctive experience. It is a more complex form in which difference is recognized and then discounted.

While Generational Intelligence places particular emphasis on the relative ability of social actors to place themselves in the position of other generations, Mannheimian perspectives appear relatively unconcerned with these issues. Rather, other generations, and here we are speaking principally about preceding generations, are perceived to be the raw material for future progress and as social entities that one defines oneself in relation to. Older generations appear, in other words, as a means to the development of separate identities. They provide the restraining other that makes one conscious of the need for social change. But there is little consideration of whether one's perception of the other is accurate or the degree to which understanding of the age-other is necessary or indeed desirable. The focus is on the way in which replacing the generational predecessor generates a sort of cultural filtering through the priorities of the emerging generation, a jettisoning of outmoded cultural baggage and the development of new social constructs for novel circumstances.

The use of generational habitus, while taking a different route, further eclipses intergenerational empathy. One's habitus is relatively free from any single location, and as suggested by Gilleard and Higgs (2005) allows relatively free-floating 'cultures of ageing' to emerge. The elective quality of these cultures, that one can effectively choose which lifestyle to adopt, contributes to the second form of closure, through the hypothesized 'blurring' of generational differences. Gilleard and Higgs (2005) argue that generations no longer make sense as fixed forms, such as kin or historical cohort, rather they should be thought of as part of a wider assemblage of options. They suggest that we are now dealing with 'post genera-tional fields' that are 'No longer confined to, nor defined by, any particular cohort or generational unit'(2005: 98). This approach solves the problem of genera-tional relations, by effectively making distinctions that are specific to generations disappear.

Solidarity and Generational Intelligence

In contrast to the predominantly European debate on generational conflict, Bengt-son and his associates (Bengtson and Putney, 2006; Lowenstein, 2007; Giarrusso *et al.*, 2005) have argued strongly for a solidarity position. Solidarity, it is claimed is the 'default' position for intergenerational relations and arises from the family, where family members generally have positive emotional bonds with one another. These bonds ensure that support is offered between generations, although the type of support will vary depending upon the generations and ages involved. This coun-ter argument is, then, based on intergenerational relations within families which it is assumed, have a profound influence on wider social attitudes.

The solidarity position draws support from the long-standing observation that judgements towards older adults are likely to be more positive in the private sphere than in the public (Biggs, 1989; Irwin, 1998). This can be characterized as the 'grandmother effect'. In other words, on balance one is likely to feel more positively towards ones' own grandmother than to 'older people' or 'the elderly' as portrayed in the popular press or political discourse (Hendricks, 2004). A simple associative exercise with a class of students can generate quite different descriptions if you ask them to describe 'old people' as compared to 'an older person that you know' (Biggs, 1992). That the grandparent as an archetypal elder figures strongly in solidarity discourse, and in the minds of younger research-ers of old age, is instructive here. It often feels that one can get on better with one's grandparental than one's parental generation: the feelings, memories and associations are less intense (Harper, 2005). They are less emotionally present, in a psychodynamic sense, and one does not, at least within the contemporary North American and Northern European model, define one's emerging adult self in opposition to the habits and restrictions of the grandparental, as compared to the parental home.

Bengtson and Putney take the family solidarity argument into this wider, pub-lic sphere by pointing to its functional value. It acts, they claim, to hold inter-generational relations together by avoiding conflict and thereby stabilizing otherwise volatile social systems. Intergenerational solidarity within families they argue: 'may hold the key to resolving these issues. This is because the essential characteristics of multigenerational families –relatedness, interdependence, and solidarity, and age integration – can influence and transform social practices and policies' (2006: 21).

Privileging family relations over social structures, these authors claim that relations in multigenerational families at a micro social level percolate up to have a 'profound but unrecognized' effects on age-relations at the macro level, which can be used by governments to make decisions about resourcing the needs of different age-groups.

Solidarity, then, becomes the personal and social ideal type that teeters between scientific research and social expectation. As part of this argument, the family is elevated to the principal solution for wider social cohesion between generations, and tacitly, as a means of reducing claims on 'scarce government resources'. However, this position has not been without its critics. Marshall *et al.* (1993) have argued that the solidarity position presupposes its own conclusions. Connidis and McMullin (2002) have pointed out that gendered power relations are not taken into account, while Lorenz-Meyer (2001) has drawn attention to the negative effects of family solidarity in maintaining social inequality between families through lineage and inheritance. The approach has little to say about people without families, and that the family retains its long-standing title as the principal sight of interpersonal violence and mistreatment across the life course (Kingston, and Penhale, 1995). Further, solidarity in the private sphere shows little evidence of mitigating social ageism in public (Bytheway, 2005) which might be expected if the solidarity hypotheses were having an effect. Rather, it replaces one form of favouritism, based on age with another based on nepotism. At the same time it is in danger of letting state responsibility for older citizens off the hook, reinforcing coercive notions of family obligation. These criticisms would lend credence to the view that rivalry between generations is tacit but deep-seated. While there is a tradition, mostly in North America, to see intergenerational relations situated in family settings and as consisting of degrees of solidarity, the substrate of intergenerational rivalry and age prejudice, appears also to be widespread. And it has been suggested that societies historically without developed welfare safety-nets would tend to eulogize the family as a haven in an otherwise harsh world (Biggs, 2007). While Giarrusso *et al.* (2005) have claimed, somewhat strangely, that conflict is actually a subcategory of solidarity, solidarity is clearly proposed as an antidote to generational conflict, without detailed consideration of the roots of such conflict.

Solidarity, conflict and binary oppositions

Under such conditions, polarized between conflict and solidarity, it is important that we move away from discourses, in policy, practice and research that simply champion one side of an argument over another. The conflict model points towards irreconcilable differences of interest between generational groups. By contrast, the solidarity position paints a world in which intergenerational relations are at root unproblematic. From the perspective of Generational Intelligence, both are only intergenerational in so far as the relationship between generations is seen as consisting, at root, of binary opposites. Relationships can, according to these two discourses, either be conflictual or based on solidarity, whereas our everyday experience tells us that often feelings towards other people, including the age-other are often more emotionally complicated. It is continually surprising how far the analysis of intergenerational relations within this binary debate returns to the expansion of only one generational position in what is a shared generational context. Thus 'generational consciousness' leans towards the triumph of the younger generation, while 'solidarity' at least with respect to adult relations champions family care for older generations. The oppositional element of such thinking takes at least three binary forms; either one is in conflict or solidarity, either one sees one side of a generational divide or the other, plus either one believes in the primacy of cohort or family as the core site of generational relations. Generational consciousness in particular, says little about a relative ability to act with awareness of one's generational circumstances as they pertain to other generational groups. The principal solution of generational consciousness is to eliminate parts of the older generation that hold the younger one back. It is not learning from, it is not learning with, rather the preceding generation is only a solution in so far as it steps aside. The solidarity position is somewhat different as it privileges one location, the family, as the most important meaning for generations, without recognizing that experience contains an amalgam of different forms of generationality. It also values solidarity over other emotional responses to the age-other, which significantly oversimplifies most people's lived experience and fails to resolve its conceptual resistance to forms of rivalry and conflict. Conceptually speaking, the binary opposition between conflict and solidarity remains in place. Binary oppositions of this type simplify thinking and action by effectively making people choose sides. In so doing, they evacuate complexity and the need to start the difficult task of taking the other point of view into account in negotiating compromises.

By changing the conceptual territory, in this instance, by focusing on the role of empathic understanding in intergenerational relations, Generational Intelligence attempts to move the debate away from the ascendancy of one cohort or one location (the family), and asks how likely is it that one can put oneself in the place of the other, rather than subsist exclusively within any one system. This is seen as furthering movement away from the simplification of intergenerational relationships painted by social ageism. Whereas the concepts of social ageism and generational consciousness focus on interests within generations and solidarity attempts to replace this evaluation with a competing normative judgement, Generational Intelligence would suggest a search for spaces where both responses can be thought, felt and contained, and relationships be consciously negotiated. It is to that question that we now turn.

5 Generational strategies and negotiation

Summary

The processes of social ageism and oppositional thinking outlined in the previous chapter raise the question of how spaces can be created that allow reflection and negotiated solutions to take place. In order to begin this search, it is important to move from an immersive state, where social assumptions about age and generation are taken for granted and the superiority of one's own generational position is assumed; to a more complex state of mind in which multiple perspectives can be recognized. Here, two elements of the process of creating positive generational distance are explored. First, it is argued that the ambiguity of intergenerational relationships has to be acknowledged, as well as its emotionally charged twin, ambivalence. Second, the presence of power imbalances between generational groups, either interpersonally or systemically, creates a situation of social masking, which can be used to protect the self and to connect to other people. These two forms of distance contribute to the creation of intergenerationally intelligent spaces, where conflicting emotions can be contained and links made to members of other groups.

Key points

- One element of generationally intelligent activity would be to keep seemingly incompatible thoughts and feelings in mind at the same time.
- Containing the desire for both solidarity and conflict in the same space avoids getting trapped in either one position and allows critical distance to develop.
- Recognizing ambivalence allows sustainable generational relations to take shape.
- In intergenerational encounters, people use a social mask or masquerade to both protect themselves and to connect to others.
- Generationally intelligent value and action positions facilitate strategies that create sustainable relations between age-groups.

Introduction

In the previous chapter, a number of barriers to intergenerational empathy were explored. A reliance on social ageism or a retreat into binary oppositions such as conflict or solidarity, can be seen as forms of simplification which make it easier to maintain a generationally 'simple state of mind'. Phenomenologically speaking, this would be experienced as an immersion within one's own generational world-view, using the mechanism of assimilation to incorporate alternative perspectives. The reduction of more complicated thoughts and feelings into binary opposites would work to neutralize any sense of ambiguity and ambivalent feelings living within an intergenerational encounter, and as such also reduce the likelihood that these dominant discourses would be challenged.

Two forms of complexity will be examined in more detail here, together with the strategies that they suggest. The first concerns the role ambiguity and ambivalence, and the argument that finding a space where multiple aspects of generational identity can be recognized and critically assessed is a key element in fostering generationally intelligent solutions. The second form of complexity involves a way in which individuals negotiate environments where parts of the self are subjected to negative evaluation. Here, the role of impression management, social masking and masquerade will be explored. The role of masquerade as a means of both connecting and protecting the self may play a particularly important role in negotiating such complexity. A third form of complexity, which saturates the others, is the possibility of a mismatch between personal generational awareness and social expectation, be this in terms of cohort culture, family roles or existential life-priorities or the interaction between them. Each form will then contribute to a consideration of how sustainable intergenerational relations might be built. In so doing, we will approach the twin steps of considering value statements and of intergenerational action.

It follows that intergenerational ambiguity can present itself in a number of ways. These include the multiple nature of generation itself and that at an everyday level, it is experienced as an amalgam of influences arising from cohort, family and life-cycle positions that depend upon context for salience. Also, the coexistence of two dominant discourses, namely those that emphasize conflict between generations and those that emphasize solidarity, which implies a value-based distinction between negative and positive forms of intergenerational activity. Because intergenerational relations are more often than not played out against a backdrop of negative stereotyping, the presentation of self is not straightforward and introduces another layer of ambiguity provoking but also generated by social masking and masquerade. Ambiguity can arise from a number of sources, including a mismatch between a person's experience of self and social attitudes towards generational location, the blurring of traditional life-stages or a tendency to eclipse the implications of dependency and infirmity in deep old age. Ambiguity shifts into the emotionally charged arena of ambivalence when there is a mismatch between generational personal perspectives and social expectations. Indeed, the very act of discovering complexity itself can provoke negative reactions, shading from avoidance into downright intolerance. As the structured life-course evolves into more ambiguous forms, ambivalence arguably becomes both a challenge and a source of more developed understanding.

Engaging with ambiguity and ambivalence

One social thinker who has shown a continuing interest in how ambiguity shades into ambivalence is Bauman (1991; 1995; 1997; 2003). He sees ambivalence as being closely tied to uncertainty and anxiety generated by contemporary societies, which as a way of re-establishing certainty divides the world into opposites. In his early work, he was particularly concerned with the division of the world into friends and enemies (Bauman, 1991) and the ambiguous nature of the stranger, who is neither, yet potentially both. Such figures, he argues, tap into a deep-seated fear of indetermination, which, because it threatens cognitive clarity and behavioural certainty, at best presents annoyance and at worst, danger. He parallels Jung (1931) in linking binary oppositions to the creation of a shadow self, where one stores, as far away as is possible things in the self that one does not want to be. Things that do not fit, produce a combination of nearness and remoteness, an 'opposition, born of the horror of ambiguity, becomes the main source of ambivalence' (Bauman, 1991: 151).

Old age, whereby as De Beauvoir reminds us, we are made strangers to ourselves (1970), would seem to be an example of such strangeness, which affects both societal reactions and personal identity. The perception of the age-other as in some way alien is increased by changed priorities between the first and second halves of adult life, changes in appearance and capacity, and negative stereotyping.

The dominant societal reaction to these forms of ambivalence, is, according to Bauman (1991), to engage in acts of assimilation which are intended to discredit and disempower any alternative possibilities. In Bauman, ambiguity and ambivalence provoke assimilative intolerance. In terms of generational relations, this can perhaps be seen in the goals associated with generational consciousness. Acting with awareness of one's own generational circumstances, is the strong suit, the ideal type for generational consciousness and a generation that becomes consciously aware of itself as a social or historical force and acts on that basis, is the endpoint of that thesis. The accumulated cultural knowledge of preceding generations are seen as a sort of rag-bag, which when sifted through, and accepted or rejected depending upon the requirements of the new. Similarly, the promotion of 'productive ageing', that social inclusion can be obtained through work and work-like activity (such as volunteering), has the generational disadvantage of colonizing the priorities of older generations with the existential tasks of younger ones. It solves the problem of social exclusion by extending working life almost indefinitely, without taking changed existential priorities into account. However, it can also put generational groups in competition for the same social roles and rewards. Both generational consciousness and productive ageing, as recipes for intergenerational relations, assimilate one set of generational priorities into another, while discounting any intrinsic qualities that the assimilated group might have.

Bauman, in 1997, proposes that recognizing and containing such ambivalence is key to contemporary moral behaviour, and elsewhere argues that

> Responsibility for the other is shot through with ambivalence: It has no obvious limits, nor does it easily translate into practical steps to be taken or refrained from – each such step being instead pregnant with consequences that are notoriously uneasy to predict and even less easy to evaluate in advance.
>
> (Bauman, 1995: 2)

He goes on to claim that 'relationships are perhaps the most common, acute, deeply felt and troublesome incarnations of ambivalence' (2003: viii).

Under such circumstances; where a phenomenon that is not obviously contained, yet where one wishes not to slip back to one or other end of a binary contradiction; it requires the simultaneous holding in mind of two seemingly incompatible aspects of the same. In other words, it is necessarily to act knowingly, or 'intelligently' by being open to the possibility that one can feel both conflict and solidarity, love and hate, be active and passive, and in different contexts, be both young and old relative to the age-other. In intergenerational situations, ambivalence has been defined by Lueseher and Pillemer (1998) as 'designate contradictions in relationships between parents and adult offspring that cannot be reconciled', and more recently as simply 'the simultaneous existence of positive and negative sentiments in the older parent–adult child relationship' (Pillemer *et al.*, 2007: 775). Pillemer *et al.* (2007) point to a number of sources of complexity in intergenerational contexts, including multiple relationships within families, status attainment, dependency and interdependency, similarity as well as difference. They maintain that all parent–child relationships are inevitably ambivalent, in so far as they contain multiple combinations of positive and negative feelings. Connidis and McMullin (2002b) explain ambivalence as 'structurally created contradictions that are made manifest in interaction' and 'simultaneously held opposing feelings or emotions that are due in part to countervailing expectations about how individuals should act' (2002b: 558). Ambivalence, in the sense of an ability to handle complexity, to think about multiple influences and recognize competing emotions, offers a phenomenological insight that is compatible with a process of emerging Generational Intelligence. And while both Lueseher and Pillemer (1998) and Bengtson *et al.* (2002) recognize the possibility of indecision and even paralysis arising from an ambivalent position, it also allows self-conscious action in so far as the complexity of mixed feelings can be overtly recognized. As such, it offers a mature step towards acknowledging a more complex world of multiple perspectives and an emotional ambiguity which requires understanding (Biggs, 2007).

Bauman (2003) following Heidegger, points out that things reveal themselves to consciousness in proportion to the frustration that they cause. In this light, it is interesting to observe that Harreveld *et al.* found ambivalence to be 'experienced as being particularly unpleasant when the ambivalent attitude holder is confronted with the necessity to a choice concerning the ambivalent attitude object' (2009: 45). Phillips *et al.* (2010) outline a number of sources of ambivalence associated with later life, including when individuals wish to be autonomous, yet are becoming dependent on others, losses of physical autonomy, a tension between volition and sense of obligation in caring contexts and roles that are incompatible with personal needs such as being both a worker and a carer. When incongruent components of an attitude surface, accompanied by feelings of uncertainty, Harreveld *et al.* (2009) report that not only does the situation become associated with negative emotion, but any anticipation of such situations does as well. Ambivalence, they report, can occur within emotional or cognitive responses, or between ideas and emotions themselves. When these positive and negative components are simultaneously available, ambivalence is experienced as unpleasant.

While Katz *et al.* (2004) have shown that care for an older relative can generate tension between independence and dependency, Lowenstein (2007) indicates that in some cases such relations can generate both high solidarity and high levels of conflictual behaviour: one only argues, perhaps, because one cares. Gaalen *et al.* (2010) found that approximately half the high contact intergenerational ties from their study, showed signs of both ambivalence and a high quality of interaction between adult children and their parents. A creative use of ambivalence may not, then, simply imply 'sitting on the fence' and a refusal to commit. It may equally generate a withholding of judgement and a tolerance of ambiguity until a more complex level of problem-solving arises.

Ambivalence and Generational Intelligence

Once an age-other has been identified, the question of how one relates to them becomes an issue. How does one evaluate the relationship, does it occasion rivalry and conflict, solidarity and common cause, or mixed feelings? Mixed feelings suggest a more complex position in which the actors recognize ambivalence. Rather than wholeheartedly and probably unreflectively liking or disliking the age-other, both emotions need to be dealt with within the same space. This highlights the degree to which actors and groups behave as if they are immersed in their own group-specific form of generational consciousness as compared to more complex forms that include an openness to multiple generational perspectives. With Generational Intelligence, ambiguity and ambivalence are turned back onto such opposites to unpack the simplifications they impose on intergenerational relations. In so doing, intergenerational relations are aligned with other forms of contemporary relationship, which, according to Smart (2000) require 'coming to terms with contingency and ambivalence as permanent and omnipresent features of modernity, as intrinsic features providing opportunities rather than signs of failure'. Seeing ambivalence as an opportunity for a deeper and sustainable set of intergenerational relations is, we would argue, key to their successful strategizing and negotiation. In sum, ambivalence need not lead to paralysis, or a retreat into over hasty action and rigid thinking. Rather, holding seemingly incompatible desires together in mind at once, and in understanding them, high levels of Generational Intelligence promise action with maturity. In so doing, it offers a mechanism that potentially contains contradictory processes. It offers a step towards acknowledging a more complex world of multiple perspectives and emotional resilience. It is in this sense that ambivalence supplies a mechanism by which sophisticated intergenerational solidarity can be maintained. For in order to create a sustainable relationship between potentially conflicting generational groups, mixed feelings need to be acknowledged and negotiated.

Negotiating protection and connection

The more complex the relationship between age identities and the perception of similarity and difference based on age, the more the social presentation of self needs to be negotiated. Questions of masquerade and the self-conscious portrayal of identity have increasingly been used in gerontological literature to examine the interaction between the social and personal experience of later life (Jung, 1931/1967; Featherstone and Hepworth, 1989; Hepworth, 2004; Woodward, 1991; 1995; Biggs, 1993; 1999; 2004; Ballard *et al.*, 2005).

The concept of a social mask, or persona, was first used by the analytic psychologist C. G. Jung to describe the way that people conform to social expectations.

> The persona is a complicated system of relations between individual consciousness and society, fittingly enough a kind of mask, designed on the one hand to make a definite impression upon others and on the other to conceal the true nature of the individual.
>
> (1931/1967, 7: 303)

At first, the persona is embraced and experimented with. As it helps the emerging adult identity find an acceptable place in the social world, one dominant persona is adopted, so much so, that over time it becomes fixed and indistinguishable from who individuals think they are. By midlife, Jung argues, this fixed position has become increasingly difficult to maintain. Within the Jungian model, because the persona is associated with social conformity, it is viewed as something that has to be outgrown if a deeper sense of personal identity is to emerge. This outgrowing becomes part and parcel of the process of individuation that takes place during midlife transitions into the second half of adult life. 'Fundamentally' Jung says, 'The persona is nothing real, it is a compromise between individual and society as to what man should appear to be' (1931/1967, 7: 158).

However, since these early days, Woodward (1991) and Biggs (1993) have revised the view of social masking in later life.

'Masquerade has to do with concealing something and presenting the very conditions of that concealment. A mathematics of difference is posited between the two terms – an inside and an outside, with the outside disguising what is within' (Woodward, 1991: 148).

Woodward (1991) argues that masquerade is used to disguise socially damaging aspects of ageing, which nevertheless reveals old age to younger generations. The pretence, however, allows access to social life and is generally accepted as a form of social coping. Biggs (1993; 1999) has emphasized that, rather than discarding the social mask with increasing maturity, the older adult learns to use it not only to protect aspects of self-development that do not fit dominant discourses on ageing and intergenerational relations, but also as a means of connection. The connective role allows a bridge to be built between the internal world of the self and other people, thus easing intergenerational interaction.

Adult ageing and intergenerational contact contain elements that are both threatening and encouraging to experiments with identity in later life. Ageing individuals simultaneously encounter two possibilities. Increased lifestyle choice holds out the promise of a flexible and potentially ageless identity (Featherstone and Hepworth, 1989). This coexists with the discovery of greater personal potential that might need to be protected from an often hostile and fragmentary social environment (Bytheway, 2005). Under such conditions, generational encounters can become a balancing act between these possibilities.

There are at least two interpretations of masquerade in later life. The 'mask of ageing' position (Featherstone, and Hepworth, 1989; Hepworth 2004), holds that the ageing body becomes a cage from which a younger self-identity cannot escape. Here, the mask motif and the problem of ageing are couched in terms of a tension between the ageing body and a youthful 'inner' self. The body, whilst it is malleable, can still provide access to a variety of consumer identities. However, as ageing gathers pace, this option becomes increasingly difficult and the body becomes a cage, which both itself entraps and, denies access to that world of choice. An endgame emerges with older people being at war with themselves, an internalized battle between a desire to express oneself and the ageing body. Ageing, as a mask, thus becomes a nightmare for the consumer dream as ageing reverses its libertarian possibilities. The mask emerges as a contradiction between the fixedness of the body and the fluidity of social images. The view that a masquerade can be used to protect a mature identity in the context of an increasingly ambiguous external environment provides an alternative strategy (Woodward, 1991; 1995; Biggs, 1993; 2004). Here, masquerade consists of language games, body language and forms of personal adornment which contribute to performances of particular versions of the self. Masquerade is of particular interest because it occurs at the meeting point of both personal identity and social appearance. It is, in this sense, deployed strategically as a bridge between inner and outer worlds. An element of social protection occurs for parts of the self that cannot be easily expressed due to contemporary expectations around age. At the same time, the experience of a long life and the existential questions that ageing brings with it are conceived as provoking an expanded and more grounded sense of self. This new and evolving self-discovery, which can be called maturity, or the 'Mature Imagination' (Biggs, 1999) has, then, to negotiate conditions that exist in a predominantly ageist society. Under circumstances of power imbalance between generations, masquerade is seen as a means of protecting this mature self from external attack, which nevertheless offers a strategy for self-expression.

Deploying social masking in such a way provides a means of negotiating identity between people of different ages as it becomes both a bridge and a shield between internal psychological and external social realities. So, relationships underscored by age can provoke a strategy which holds a more positive and protective nuance than Jung's or Featherstone and Hepworth's interpretations would suggest. Using a masquerade in this way is seen to be a result of an irony of later life: that an increase in complex understanding and an increase in negative social coercion are experienced simultaneously. Rather than simply being the sum of attributes through which a sense of identity can be deduced, masquerade becomes a means by which an active agent negotiates the intergenerational environment.

There is an increasing body of literature suggesting that older adults, rather than becoming fixed in their social strategies, have developed complex skills for intergenerational negotiation and self-presentation. Holstein and Gubrium (2000) show that in interview situations, older respondents are adaptive and responsive to the expectations and ground-rules of an interview, taking care to generate appropriate communication. Williams and Nussbaum (2001), drawing on an extensive programme of research, points to the potential for misunderstanding between generations and the tendency for older adults to use more complex communication strategies than other age-groups. Hummert *et al.* (1994) report the use of communication strategies aimed at interrupting negative feedback cycles such as age stereotypes in interpersonal communication. Communications by older adults were seen to be both complex and to include a mixture of positive and negative attributions. Grenier (2007) suggests that crossing age and generational boundaries can hold the potential for both connection and conflict: that emotional connection across a sense of being an insider or an outsider to the feelings generated by age difference provokes negotiation, both in interaction with helping professional and in intergenerational research. Stuifbergen *et al.* (2008) point to the need for complex family relations to be negotiated and that a resulting good parent–adult-child relationship was a much stronger motivator for giving support than a sense of obligation. Van den Hoonaard (2009) when examining self-representation in later life, found that widowers used a number of strategies to affirm their masculinity. A somewhat overbearing emphasis on managing what the female interviewer identifies as a 'real man' position, arise, she argues, in compensation for threats arising from an absence of components of that identity, including a heterosexual relationship, employment and youthful vigour. Nikander (2009) found that baby boomers deployed a 'provisional continuity device' a strategy that enabled speakers to simultaneously acknowledge and distance themselves from life-course change, while Norrick (2009) found the construction of multiple identities, with narrators telling stories about themselves that included sometimes contradictory positions, as well as taking the perspectives of others into account. What older adults revealed and how they reflected on such contents were used by listeners to form an opinion about the teller and their current identity. Coupland (2009) discusses the importance of changing strategies in midlife and later life towards the body and what she calls the reversibility of ageing as ageing identities are commodified in popular culture. This work is similar to that of Clarke and Griffin (2007) who refer to visible and invisible ageing and the role of 'beauty work' in strategizing age and appearance.

One of the ways that individuals negotiate the contradictions of contemporary ageing is through the submersion of elements of self-experience that cannot be expressed directly and be socially accepted. These elements are hidden from social view, protected in an interior world, such that social connection and conformity are separated psychologically from an inner world of self. It is within this imaginative realm, beyond the masquerade, that personal development and integration may take place, which may not be so prominent during earlier life-phases. The blurring of identities between generations, noted by Featherstone and Hepworth (1991) adds ambiguity to this situation. A broad band of activities, including the growth of retirement communities (Laws, 1997; Bernard *et al.*, 2007), consumer lifestyles (Gilleard and Higgs, 2000), and in longevity research and bio-scientific innovation (Butler *et al.*, 2008; Olshansky *et al.*, 2007), can also be interpreted as part of a process that confuses established meanings of age and generation. Here, each activity represents a social strategy of staying young or of agelessness in the face of adult ageing. The blurring consists of strategies to avoid ageing and of presenting an age-neutral lifestyle to the wider world, this results, at least in the eyes of the older parties, in a lessening of the gap between younger and older generations (Biggs *et al.*, 2007). However, consideration of the past, memory and of experience that goes beyond the here and now becomes particularly problematic once ageing has been subsumed under the persona of the happy shopper. The process of ageing, is, alternatively, of existential importance, lending depth to our understanding, if we allow it, of the wider human condition (Tornstam, 2003). On the one hand, protection is required to safeguard the self from social-cultural stereotyping that may ultimately restrict possibilities for personal growth and social inclusion. On the other, some form of connection is necessary in order to maintain social engagement, and specifically engagement with other generational groups. If this argument is accepted, then an ageing identity still has to negotiate a path between an excess of social expectation and of uncertainty. Generationally intelligent action suggest a complex world that includes protective and connective elements and cannot simply remain immersed in a single generational position to maintain a serviceable mature identity.

Strategies for Generational Intelligence

The pragmatic aspect of intergenerational relations, from the position of Generational Intelligence would be found in negotiation and the development of strategies that respond to values and actions between generations. And here two forms of negotiation have been addressed. The first involves the negotiation of contradictory positions, so that elements that at first seem to force intergenerational relations to one or other end of a set of binary opposites can be contained within the same space. This allows strategic values to develop that are not based solely on conflict or unreflective solidarity, but on a more complex and considered form that would also facilitate intergenerational communication. This requires both the recognition of difference and an ability to return to the other, now seeing them less through the lens of one's own generational position and more through seeking intergenerational consensus. While it may be difficult to fully accommodate through putting one-self completely in the shoes of the age-other, increased Generational Intelligence generates the possibility of a space in which multiple generational perspectives can be given voice, allowing forms of compromise to emerge that take elements of each position into account. The second form of negotiation occurs through the use of intergenerational strategies that both protect and connect. The deployment of a social masquerade, in conditions often not of one's own choosing, offers a more complex presentation of self when intergenerational relationships are being negotiated. It identifies a tension between protection and connection that needs to be consciously considered. This strategy protects aspects of self-development that are threatened by age-stereotyping, and forms a bridge to others that may live with different generational priorities, but nevertheless present the prospect of finding common ground. Recognizing ambivalence and ambiguity, through negotiation allows a more complex and nuanced understanding of intergenerational relations to emerge. Both open a critical distance between thought and activity. Neither is immersive, and as such present a space for a deeper appreciation of the self, of age-others and a measured response to intergenerational relations. Taken together, they offer a way of negotiating ambiguous value systems and a way of engaging in ambivalent intergenerational action.

Beyond generational categories, toward Generational Intelligence

Generational Intelligence attempts to move beyond bipolarities of conflict or solidarity, in terms of process, while at the same time recognizing that as part of the gerontological project, it has to take a position, in Taylor's (1989) sense, that in the process of articulating claims implicit in our actions, we need also to become sure of the place on which we make our stand. Generational Intelligence does not argue for an 'age neutral' or 'age-irrelevant' society, however, but for a negotiation of generation specific needs and goals. This process would take into account steps towards Generational Intelligence that arise from considerations of the dimensions of self-awareness and generational empathy. It also examines the contested, yet ultimately positive strength of ambiguity and ambivalence in intergenerational relations, that both gives rise to and help to contain and make manageable tensions in the experience of self and of other.

   In terms of generationally intelligent action, low levels of Generational Intelligence may result in intergenerational relations that do not take multiplicity into account and thereby, act out one pole or another as if it were the only and natural way to behave. A middle level would include awareness of conflicting alternatives, but without a clearly articulated understanding of generational influences, lead to psychological paralysis and inaction or behavioural avoidance. A high-level response would keep alternatives simultaneously within the same mental space, so that the intergenerational participant can act with both in mind. The journey from unself-conscious immersion to generationally intelligent action, is part of an emerging critical distance between self and other that allows experiment with alternative generational strategies to take place. Previously fixed positions then have the chance of becoming one of a variety of alternative styles of engagement. Concepts common in the literature, describing conflict solidarity and ambivalence, each referring to life-course, lineage or cohort contexts, could then be thought of as strategies that are adopted towards intergenerational relationships, rather than embedded characteristics. This would constitute a significant step, not only to empathic understanding, but also the creation of mutually compatible intergenerational activities.

When the recognition of mixed feelings and social performances are put together, they not only make a link between ambivalence and social strategies, they also allow a different way of thinking about the relationship between ambiguity, ambivalence and solidarity between generations. Being able to tolerate ambiguity, for example between attitudes arising from cohort experience, family position and one's current place in the life course. Being able to create a space that can contain ambivalent thoughts and feelings, for example about independence and dependency, autonomy and interdependence. Both of these abilities, developing as forms of Generational Intelligence would form the processes by which solidarity between generations can be sustained. Rather than seeing family solidarity, for example as a cultural given, it would now be the behavioural consequence of a series of social and historical processes. Its value lies in the degree to which it builds toward long-term intergenerational negotiation and allows enough flexibility as circumstances develop over time.

6   Generations and family

Summary

The goal of this chapter is to examine and understand how increased life expectancy, demographic shifts and changes in family structures combined with societal changes affect relationships between different family generations. Recognition of these changes and flexibility in adapting to them might be crucial for creating solidarity in intergenerational family relations. Such an understanding is related to the view that the couple and family orientation of social life and the value attached to sociability make the family a main reference point in the ageing process.

Key implications of this transformation are a new architecture for social and familial relations. This has a direct bearing on the meaning of generations and generational relationships within families, as families are multigenerational by definition. Even ties between siblings, members of the same generation, begin because they share the same parents.

In this chapter, we consider the implications of the aforementioned changes for different family generations, within the theoretical frameworks of the life-course, intergenerational solidarity-conflict and intergenerational ambivalence perspectives. We will look at the intersection of the public and private spheres and how it affects grasping the meaning of generation and impacts intergenerational family relations. How these relations could be negotiated within different families in various cultures and between different generations in a family.

Such a discussion will enrich and extend the knowledge base on how families in the twenty-first century will meet the challenges of global ageing and how they can place themselves in the position of different family generations. We suggest that Generational Intelligence (Gen I) is an important mechanism in facilitating adaptation to these societal and familial changes and enhancing intergenerational family relations.

Key points

- the effect of global ageing and societal changes on intergenerational family relations;

- • the meaning of changing family structures on behaviours, roles and family relations;
- • analyzing the usefulness of different theoretical perspectives, i.e. life-course intergenerational family solidarity-conflict and intergenerational ambivalence, for understanding the meaning of generations and family relations;
- • examining the intersection between the public and private spheres and its impact on family relations;
- • looking at the implications of developing a mechanism of Generational Intelligence and how a high Gen I can facilitate fruitful negotiations between different family generations.

Global ageing and changing family structures

Rarely have societies witnessed a 'silent revolution' of such significance as the global phenomenon of population ageing (Kinsella, 2000) which impacts family generational relationships and changes the landscape of families. During the last decades, there has been unprecedented growth in the number and proportion of older persons in most countries around the world, a trend which is expected to continue. This reflects a 'globalization' of ageing, even though the pace is more gradual in some countries and more rapid in others (Bengtson *et al.*, 2003; Kinsella, 2000). The proportion of people aged 60 years and over is increasing faster than any other age group. In 2025, there will be a total of about 1.2 billion people 60 years and older (WHO, 2002a).

The demographic changes show that more people spend more years within family structures, but that these structures are constantly changing. Moreover, population ageing and increased life expectancy adds to the diversity and complexity of family lives and intergenerational bonds (Lowenstein, 2007).

Bengtson (2001) distinguishes two levels of analysis, the micro (private sphere) and macro (public sphere). The micro level pertains to exchanges among family members, like among children, parents and grandparents. The macro refers to relationships between cohorts that are often defined in terms of specific events, national or global, like in the US, the baby boomers. It is, thus, important to learn how generations are defined within these two spheres and how they intersect and impact intergenerational family relations. In this chapter and the one that follows on caregiving issues, we will attempt to unpack this topic.

Diversity of families

Along with population ageing, marked changes are evident in family structures. There has been a sharp decline in fertility, changes in the timing of family transitions, increased rates of divorce and changes in family structures from pyramids to 'beanpoles' with an increased availability of extended, intergenerational kin as family resources (Bengtson, 2001). Changes in patterns of family formation and dissolution and the ensuing diversification of families and households might lead to more complex and 'atypical' household formations. This diversity is related to what Stacey (1990) labelled the postmodern family, characterized by 'structural fragility' and a greater dependence on the voluntary commitment of its members (Lowenstein, 2005), which creates uncertainty in intergenerational relations (Lowenstein *et al.*, 2008). Such uncertainty is closely related to the ability of a family and its members to successfully negotiate intergenerational family relations.

Improvements in life expectancy that allow parents to see their children age through adulthood and their grandchildren form new families of their own (Silverstein and Marenco, 2001) is evidence to the growing complexity of the relations between different generations within a family context today. It also means that intergenerational family relations can serve as important sources of support, especially in times of transitions or acute emotional or practical need.

Hagestad and Uhlenberg (2006) argue that global ageing will promote age integration in intergenerational family relations. The circumstances where multiple family generations share several decades together promotes interdependencies between family generations, what they term 'linked lives' (Elder, 1994; Hagestad, 2003). For example, when adult children become parents their parents will acquire an additional role in their familial life – that of a grandparent. The importance of the extended versus the nuclear family is evidenced by data which show that in the US in the 1970s 40 per cent of families were nuclear, whereas in 2000 this figure was less than 25 per cent (Williams *et al.*, 2005). Increased rates of divorce and delayed timing of parenthood, though, might have a negative impact on intergenerational family relationships (Szinovacz, 2007). However, Logan and Spitze (1996) and Bengtson (2001) suggested that such factors may have heightened the salience of parent–child relationships and those of extended family relations as the most enduring relations.

Thus, demographic change and the increased duration of family ties across several generations motivate the study of intergenerational family relationships (Bengtson and Lowenstein, 2003). Family life, on the one hand, offers many potential benefits. Families can provide some goods and services more efficiently than individuals or markets (Daatland and Lowenstein, 2005). Families may resolve differences among members and help negotiate compromises better than other groups where family members care about one another, know each other well, have long-term commitments to each other (Bengtson, 2001) and share a common set of values or understanding of their obligations to one another (Lowenstein and Daatland, 2006). There are also potential costs to family life, arising from compromises because individual family members have different preferences and needs (Phillips *et al.*, 2010).

Understanding how individuals within families coordinate and make decisions and how they negotiate compromises and trade the perceived costs and benefits (now and in the future) of different choices about family life, lies at the heart of our attempt to better understand intergenerational family relations by introducing the conceptual framework of Gen I, where acquiring a high GI might facilitate successful negotiations between family members.

We will attempt to deal with the following questions: how does longevity affect family life when four generations may be alive at the same time? How does the perception that life is long affect decisions about investments in children and grandchildren and expectations in each generation about providing and receiving help at different life stages. What are the unique features of family as an institution that coordinates the sometimes conflicting goals of individuals? Do families have unique ways of resolving conflicts and enhancing benefits of family membership? How do norms and other aspects of the social and economic context affect choices and the process by which families make choices?

Accordingly, the chapter includes four parts: First, a brief review of intergenerational family relations – the definition of a family, its salience and the nature and extent of intergenerational familial ties. Second, outlining main theoretical frameworks in this area of research. Third, discussing the meaning of generations within the private and public spheres and the interconnectedness between them. Finally, the implications of Generational Intelligence for understanding families and generations.

Family intergenerational relations

Within social structures, the family is located somewhere at the centre, below the public-collective sphere but above the individual system. The family holds a crucial position at the intersection of a number of categories like generational lines and gender. Data show that because individuals live longer and share more years and experiences with other generations, intergenerational bonds among adult family members may be even more important than in earlier decades (Bengtson *et al.*, 1995; Bengtson, 2001). However, families in the twenty-first century are also entering into new intergenerational caring relations with regard to intensity and duration, necessitating a renegotiation of relationships (Biggs and Lowenstein, forthcoming). Some of these renegotiations might lead to conflicts and even to abusive situations, unless there is a successful process of negotiation and renegotiation.

The modern family, as opposed to the traditional one, according to Durkheim (1933) is a family of relationships, more 'centered on people rather than things', having to assure for each of its members, young and old, women and men, the conditions for the construction of his/her personal and social identity. Although the notion of identity has basically evolved as a socio-psychological concept related to the self, groups such as the family may also have an identity (Lowenstein, 2003) as do larger groups such as cohorts or nations. When a group, like the family, recognizes and behaves on the basis of a shared identity, a generation can then become a motor for social changes. The family acts as an enfolding network that distances within-group relationships from external threat. Additionally, the social gerontological perspective emphasizes the protective value of generations through care relations and reciprocity (Lowenstein *et al.*, 2007; 2008). However, if such an identity is diminished, family solidarity might turn disharmonious and abusive relationships might ensue.

Bourdieu's (1996) perspective on the family was based on the central themes of capital and habitus, focusing on intergenerational transmission of different types of capital between different family generations, referring to three types – economic, social and cultural: economic related to income and inheritance; social – knowledge and specific identities of individuals; cultural – embodied cultural capital. Habitus relates to the legitimation for preferences, practices and behaviours based on past experiences within the family. He characterizes the family as a specific objective and subjective social unit which organizes the way individual family members from different generations perceive social reality.

It is evident from this perspective that generational relationships are key to the analysis of social and familial dynamics. In the sequence of generations, families and societies create continuity and change with regard to parents and children, economic resources, political power and cultural hegemony. In all these spheres, generations are a basic unit of social reproduction and social change – in other words, of stability over time as well as renewal.

Family characteristics

Intergenerational family bonds reflect a diversity of forms related to *individual, familial and cohort characteristics*. These serve as markers for differences in socialization, roles, culture, values and access to resources, thereby shaping family relations and providing the ground upon which fruitful negotiations can be achieved. On the *individual level*, two variables are especially important: *age and gender (*Silverstein *et al.*, 2006). The age of family members has to be considered because age causes changes in roles and responsibilities. It places a person along various stages of the life-course either as an adolescent, middle age or old age. Age is also related to the person's position within a certain historical cohort – an example of which would be belonging to the boomer generation, which would affect attitudes to family and to younger and older age groups and sharing of economic resources within a family (Biggs, 2007). Gender is important because women and men undergo different socialization processes, and women tend more to maintain social relations between family members and are maybe better able to facilitate modes of negotiations when family conflicts arise. Women are also most likely to act as primary caregivers, even though in recent years they move more and more into the workforce (Connidis, 2001). *Family attributes* refer to positions that members hold within the family – are they married, divorced, widowed, children, parents and grandparents. The *generational organization* of the family is particularly critical for those in middle age, a phase in life when individuals are likely to play multiple roles (Evandrou and Glaser, 2004; Attias-Donfut, 2005). Thus, family structure – meaning the number of family generations, proximity between adult children and older parents – shapes opportunities for engagement, defining and reinforcing meaningful social roles and those roles that are burdensome (Silverstein *et al.*, 2006; Lowenstein *et al.*, 2008). However, the successful enactment of these roles requires a process of continual renegotiation between different family members and different generations within a family (Szinovacz, 2008).

The extension of life expectancy, means that for several decades of adulthood people have family generations above and below them with competing needs (Dykstra and Komter, 2006). Thus, in view of current demographic, socio-economic and structural changes in families, the following issues should be addressed: examining how are families adjusting intergenerational interactions and relationships given global socio-economic developments and demographic changes; exploring if the notion of family should be redefined, moving beyond the traditional definition of a nuclear or conjugal family and how would such a redefinition impact intergenerational family relations; the contribution of each individual family member to the intergenerational familial exchange and how is this performed and negotiated within the encounter impacting the process, outcome and potential for connection or conflict between generations; The differences in such patterns across various cultural and national contexts. Most of these issues are reflected in several leading theoretical traditions, as discussed in the next section.

Theoretical perspectives on intergenerational family relations

We will examine several theoretical perspectives for understanding relations between different family generations, namely, life-course, intergenerational solidarity-conflict and intergenerational ambivalence.

The life-course perspective

The tenets of the life-course approach emphasize transitions, trajectories and societal impact as key concepts (Hagestad, 2003; Lowenstein, 2003). The various life-course perspectives share the following main premises: The life-course is a social phenomenon that reflects the intersection of social, cultural and historical factors with personal biography (e. g. Elder, 1985). As Hagestad (2003) points out, families emerge as critical mediators between developing individuals and societies in flux, with Roos (2005) adding that life's turning points are seen as negative if they arise from macro social change, while personal intergenerational events are more likely to be perceived positively. Elder (1985) states that: 'Each generation is bound to the fateful decisions and events in the other's life-course' (p. 40). This is related to the concept of 'linked lives' (Hagestad, 2003) which postulates that the opportunities and constraints faced by individuals are shaped by the needs and resources of different generational family members whose lives run close to their own. In other words, people are affected by what happens to others in the family and when making decisions, they consider the consequences there might be for others. This might form a basis for successfully attaining and sustaining high Generational Intelligence. A life-course approach to family life would link three metrics of individual lifetime, social (family) time and historical time. The individual lifetime metric relates to chronological age and age stratification and the meanings, behavioural expectations and vulnerabilities associated with particular ages.

The linkage between particular age groups and family-event sequences assumes an underlying set of age and filial norms. Historical circumstances, which reflect historical time, relate to broad social and cultural changes, such as migration or economic shifts, mould and reshape mutual support within the family (Hareven, 1994; Elder and Caspi, 1990). Ethnicity and culture within these three metrics, reflecting social time which might differentially impact well-being of individuals and families who are members of different ethnic and cultural groups. It might be also differentially related to how generations negotiate family relations and relations with other cohorts in society. The approach provides a comprehensive framework for understanding familial generational relations and the influences that stabilize and lead to change over time, especially between families from different cultural groups, where different family norms and values are transmitted, what Bourdieu (1996) refers to as the social and cultural habitus.

The aforementioned three metrics of individual lifetime, social (family) time and historical time relate to three areas of generations and self outlined in Chapter 1. The individual time reflects a look at self-perceptions that are based on age, how people think about their 'travelling' through adult life and how these patterns of thought might change as they move through time and, grow older. Regarding social-family time, it is connected to the emotional figures that inhabit their world of the family, and the historical time where different existential priorities emerge as an individual progress along the life-course within a specific social context.

The varying degrees of interdependence in multigenerational exchanges during the life-course weaves a variety of dynamic macro – social-historical time – and micro – individual and social – familial threads, where the various types of habitus that Bourdieu (1996) explicated are reflected. Rather than taking one age cohort only, for example, 'youth' or 'older persons,' research and public policy should adopt an intergenerational lens to look at issues of social change, conflict and solidarity among generations in families and in societies.

The solidarity-conflict position

Several theoretical positions have been advanced to capture the complexity and multifaceted nature of intergenerational family relations in later life. Since the early 1970s, Bengtson and his colleagues have developed the intergenerational solidarity position and continued to develop and expand this model within the Longitudinal Study of Generations (LSOG) (i.e. Bengtson and Roberts, 1991; Silverstein and Bengtson, 1997; Silverstein *et al.*, 2010).

The solidarity position reflects several theoretical traditions including: (a) theories of social organization, (b) social psychology of group dynamics, and (c) family developmental perspective. The central contribution of the sociological theories of social organization to later models of solidarity lay in describing the relevant bases of group solidarity: normative perceptions internalized by group members, functional interdependencies among group members and consensus between members over rules of exchange (Roberts *et al.*, 1991). The contribution of social psychologists to the development of the intergenerational solidarity position is by extending the classic definition of consensus over rules of exchange to incorporate the notion of similarity among members of the group. Combining the classical and the social psychological definitions of family solidarity, five elements may be identified: normative integration, functional interdependence, similarity or consensus, mutual affection and interaction (Lowenstein and Katz, 2010). The sociological family perspective emphasized integration related to various dimensions: Structural integration, affectual integration, consensual integration, functional integration, normative integration and goal integration (Nye and Rushing, 1969).

The intergenerational solidarity position emerged from the aforementioned theories, as a response to concern about the isolation of the nuclear family, even though the myth about the extended families of the past was not congruent with reality. As it was found that relationships with kin in extended family is meaningful and provide support in modern times as well (Bengtson, 2001), co-residence with children in most developed societies is usually in order to answer a need of one or more of the generations, like older parents needing care (Hareven, 1994) or in immigrant families, where both adult children and older parents may need instrumental as well as emotional support (Lowenstein and Katz, 2000). But it might lead to situations where renegotiating intergenerational family relations is imperative.

Intergenerational solidarity position perceives parent–adult-child relationships as a primary source of mutual emotional and instrumental support (Bengtson *et al.*, 2000). Bengtson and Schrader (1982) defined intergenerational solidarity as a multidimensional structure and codified six principal dimensions that reflect behavioural, affectual, cognitive and structural components of the large family: the six are structural solidarity, association, functional, emotional, normative and consensus. (Roberts *et al.*, 1991). The mixed findings regarding the interrelationships of the six dimensions and their ability to explain intergenerational family relations led to the conclusion that families might develop varied patterns of intergenerational solidarity and different ways to negotiate familial relationships. For example, findings from the five nations OASIS study (Norway, Germany, UK, Spain and Israel) and from the US (based on the Longitudinal Study of Generations) reveal a four-class typology of intergenerational relations, composed of analysis of emotional closeness and conflict in family relations: the first class had high probability of affection and low probability of conflict, suggesting an *amicable* type of relationship. The second class had low likelihood of both affection and conflict, implying an emotionally *detached* type of relationship. The third class was characterized by low affection and high conflict, a type labelled as *disharmonius*. Finally, the fourth class exhibited high probabilities of affection and conflict, these opposing feelings suggesting an *ambivalent* type of relationship. There was a different distribution of the four types in the various countries related to family culture and social context (Silverstein *et al.*, 2010).

The conceptual framework of intergenerational solidarity represents one of several enduring attempts in family sociology to examine and develop a theory of family cohesion (Mancini and Blieszner, 1989).

Although the solidarity paradigm became the 'gold standard' for assessing intergenerational relations, its component dimensions were not indicative of a unitary construct (Atkinson *et al.*, 1986; Roberts and Bengtson, 1990). So does solidarity really capture today's complex and changing patterns and behaviours of different generations within the family system?

Intergenerational solidarity within families raises the question: 'How will the family group deal with differences or conflicts that arise between generations and negotiate their resolution for the betterment of individuals, families and the social order?' (Bengtson and Putney, 2006: 20). In a robust restatement of what is essentially the solidarity position, they claim:

> Intergenerational relations at the micro-social level within multigenerational families have a profound but unrecognized influence on relations between age groups at the societal level. . . . The essence of multigenerational families is interdependence between generations and its members, and this will tend to mitigate schisms between age groups over scarce government resources.
>
> (2006: 28)

It should be noted, though, as Marshall points out, that

> It should be clear that the Bengtson legacy has provided an enduring set of analytical categories to understand changes in family life in relation to aging and intergenerational relationships . . . to continue his work will require extending the concepts to accommodate the greater dispersion of members of intergenerational families and changes in the operationalization of family solidarity in a global context.
>
> (2007: 17)

The model has adapted to innovations in methods and challenges to its dominance and universality. It was modified in 1985 to become the 'solidarity-conflict' model, which incorporates conflict and focuses also on possible negative effects of too much solidarity, in other words, too much involvement of family members in each other's lives like parents trying to protect their growing up children or adult children trying to protect very frail old parents. They argue, thus, that as a normative aspect of these relations it is likely to affect the perception of relationships and willingness of family members to assist each other and renegotiate familial generational relations (Lowenstein, 2007). Conflict allows for resolving issues, thereby enhancing the overall quality of the relationship rather than harming it, and should actually be integrated into the solidarity framework (Parrott and Bengtson, 1999). However, these two dimensions of solidarity and conflict do not represent a single continuum, from high solidarity to high conflict. Rather, intergenerational family relations can exhibit both high solidarity and high conflict, or low solidarity and low conflict, depending on family dynamics, relations between generations and circumstances (Bengtson *et al.*, 2000).

Intergenerational solidarity and conflict are manifested at two different levels, as suggested by Bengtson and Murray (1993). They differentiate between the macro-public arena and the micro-intergenerational family level – the 'smaller social contract'. On the macro level, attention should be paid to the larger social context where social norms are created and activated, and where state policies and responses of various welfare regimes to the needs of the growing elderly populations are shaped. On the micro-family level, attention should be devoted to issues of filial obligations, expectations of different generations in the family and the actual flow of help and support between generations. Much of Bengtson and his associates work, though, concentrated on the family as a place where the micro and macro – the public and the private spheres interact.

In formulating the 'family solidarity-conflict' model, Bengtson and Silverstein joined a group of contemporary theorists of ageing who view conflictual relations as an important element in understanding ageing as part of a system of age stratification, where relations between different age groups are based not only on norms of reciprocity or equality of exchange. There are conflicts between generations over resources such as access to labour markets, income and occupational prestige as well as competing demands of different generations in three and four generation families.

Most of what we do know ignores the fact that family members in contemporary society may, for example, provide financial help or other assistance across three generations instead of only two, the potential for reciprocity over the long term (e.g. Lowenstein *et al.*, 2008), there is a potential for coordination but also conflict among adult siblings whose older parents need care. The concept of Gen I should, thus, be useful in a period of global ageing and changing family structures.

This begged the question of whether intergenerational family relationships that were both emotionally close and conflicted (or emotionally distant with little conflict) were meaningful and empirically discernable within the solidarity design. This impasse was bridged by parallel conceptual and empirical developments brought about by the integration of conflict within a more general approach to social cohesion and renewed interest in the concept of ambivalence. We should pay attention to parent–adult-child relations as 'networks of multiple ties and interactions with both positive and negative qualities and outcomes' (Ward, 2008: S244).

The ambivalence perspective

Modernity is characterized by the depth and pervasiveness of a 'dilemmatic' attitude namely, structural contradictions built into societal organizations that result in cognitive dilemmas at the common sense and ideological levels (Billing *et al.*, 1988). Weigert (1991) speaks of modernity in terms of pluralism and multi-valence. People in contemporary societies face a characteristically modernist dilemma: the ambiguity of competing meanings and the ambivalence of conflicting feelings.

Within the world of a family, this tension a person feels between, for example, individual and group needs, takes on special intensity. Group members seek both autonomy and personal gains that the individualistic culture holds so central, and the security and commonwealth that everyone needs and the group-family provides (Weigert, 1991). Involvement in family throughout life means that members experience loss of deep identities and the reversal of relationships of power and dependency between parents and children (Weigert and Hastings, 1977; Fingerman *et al.*, 2006). This led to the renewed interest in the concept of ambivalence.

The term ambivalence, reflecting contradictions and ambiguities in relationships, was introduced by Luescher and Pillemer (1998) as a valuable revived conceptual perspective for studying parent–child relations in later life and relations between generations in families. Luescher (2002) has proposed ambivalence as an alternative to both the solidarity and conflict perspectives to serve as a model for orienting sociological research on intergenerational relations. The term ambivalence has a relatively long history in the field of psychology, both in psychotherapy and in research on attitudes in close relationships, and in sociology it reflects postmodern approaches to family.

They proposed intergenerational ambivalence to 'designate contradictions in relationships between parents and adult offspring that cannot be reconciled' (Luescher and Pillemer, 1998: 416). The concept of ambivalence, they argue, should be the primary topic of study of intergenerational relations, since 'societies and the individuals within them are characteristically ambivalent about relationships between parents and children in adulthood' (Pillemer and Luescher, 2004: 6).

Three aspects of family life are suggested as being likely to generate ambivalence (Luescher and Pillemer, 1998: 417): (1) Ambivalence between dependence and autonomy – in adulthood the desire of parents and children for help and support and the countervailing pressures for freedom from the parent–child relationship; (2) Ambivalence resulting from conflicting norms regarding intergenerational relations – for example, conflicting norms of reciprocity and solidarity in caregiving which become problematic in situations that involve chronic stress; and (3) Ambivalence resulting from solidarity, like the 'web of mutual dependency', revealed in elder abuse case studies.

Based on his work with Pillemer, Luescher and Pillemer (1998) proposed a heuristic model which is an attempt to combine postulate of ambivalence with considerations of the two basic dimensions implied in the concept of generations. The first of these recognizes that families are institutionally embedded in pre-existing systems which include the structural, procedural and normative conditions in a society. These institutional conditions are, on the one hand, reinforced and reproduced by the way people behave. On the other, they can also be modified and can lead to innovation in family relations. Reproduction and innovation are two poles of the social field in which the family is realized as an institution. Tension between these two poles may be conceived as referring to structural ambivalence. Second, at the level of relationships, parents and children share a certain degree of similarity that is reinforced by the intimacy of mutual learning processes, and contain a potential for closeness and subjective identification. At the same time, similarity is also a cause of and reason for distancing as children strive towards developing their identity and establish their autonomy.

Ambivalence, as defined by Luescher (1999) and by Luescher and Pillemer (1998), emerges when dilemmas between positive and negative aspects of social relations and social structures are interpreted as being in contradiction. They argue that the concept of ambivalence is a good reference point because it avoids normative assumptions and moral idealizations. Moreover, it points to a pragmatic necessity for researching strategies that shape intergenerational relations, as for example, when negotiation and renegotiation are needed.

Connidis and McMullin (2002a; 2002b) propose that ambivalence can be viewed as a brokering concept between the solidarity model and the problematization of family relations, and offer a critical perspective through their work on divorce impact on intergenerational family relations. One of their central tenets is that individuals experience ambivalence when social structural arrangements frustrate their attempts to negotiate within relationships. For example, women have societal pressures to care and less opportunity to resist, despite the entry of more women into the labour force. Hence, they are more likely than men to experience ambivalence. Thus, women have to negotiate and renegotiate their care-giving situations and ambivalence created by competing demands on their time in order to manage work, family life and caring.

Given that ambivalence has its basis in the tension between autonomy and dependence, it is not surprising that intergenerational family relations are among the most ambivalent, extending well beyond the more obvious applications to adolescent children and their parents (Fingerman *et al.*, 2004). In mature parent–child relations, ambivalence levels are elevated when parental health is poor (Fingerman *et al.*, 2006; Willson *et al.*, 2003), as parents become increasingly frail and reliant on their adult children to whom they were formerly providers (Willson *et al.*, 2006).

Ambivalence vs. Solidarity-Conflict

Looking at the 'history' of the development of the renewed ambivalence perspective, it should be noted that Bengtson *et al.* (2002) criticize the ambivalence concept on several grounds.

They ask how it differs from a symbolic interactionist approach to role conflict, meaning that the suggested ambivalence perspective is actually similar to that approach, so is it really then a new approach? They also wonder how it can predict or explain intergenerational family dynamics better than their own approach, and view ambivalence as perhaps complementing the solidarity-conflict framework, which is conceptually adequate for exploring mixed feelings. They explain this proposition by claiming that 'From the intersection of solidarity and conflict comes ambivalence, both psychological and structural' (Bengtson *et al.*, 2002: 575). They argue that both the solidarity-conflict and the ambivalence models can be regarded as lenses 'through which one can look at family relationships' (p. 575).

While conflict in the solidarity paradigm was originally conceptualized as a form of 'anti-solidarity', more recent theorizing has explicitly incorporated ambivalence into the model as the space where affection and conflict intersect. Detecting ambivalence within this more general solidarity framework extended an empirical approach to the study of families that classified relationships into meaningful categories that may consist of inconsistent elements (Van Galen and Dysktra, 2006; Silverstein and Litwak, 1993; Giarrusso *et al.*, 2005). Over its historical development, the solidarity-conflict model has had as its goal to be a comprehensive, parsimonious and universal scheme for describing intergenerational family relationships. Yet, despite its widespread application, there have been few cross-national comparisons of the model. However, the recent availability of multi-national data, mostly in Europe, has provided the opportunity to explicitly test the application of the solidarity-conflict paradigm in different contexts and the potential to evaluate how families in different national contexts differ in their intergenerational ties and the way they negotiate intergenerational family relations and if they are able to achieve successful and sustainable relations, in other words having acquired a high Generational Intelligence (Lowenstein, 2007; Lowenstein *et al.*, 2007; 2008; Lowenstein and Daatland, 2006; Katz *et al.*, 2005). The results basically support the more harmonious perspective of the solidarity model which might attest to successful negotiations between generations. Conflict and ambivalence may be useful heuristically but are difficult to measure empirically and may be more prone to social desirability effects, when measured quantitatively.

The OASIS data (OASIS – Old Age and Autonomy: The Role of Service Systems and Intergenerational Family Solidarity was funded by the EU under the fifth framework programme) underscore the importance, in an intergenerational context, of individuals actively negotiating and renegotiating solutions and management strategies in response to change and transitions over the life-course (Katz *et al.*, 2005). This points again to the meaningful role of understanding different generational views and accommodating to such views when circumstances require. In other words, having a high Generational Intelligence allows to bring to fruition successful negotiations between different family generations.

These clashing positions offer different conceptual lenses for understanding the complex and diverse family relationships in societies undergoing social change and provide different ways to understand micro-level interpersonal relations and macro-level structural forces and the interactions between these levels. The clash is between the post-positivists who developed and tested the long-standing intergenerational solidarity-conflict paradigm (Bengtson and Schrader, 1982; Bengtson and Roberts, 1991; Parrott and Bengtson, 1999) and the critical theorists who advocate the revival of intergenerational ambivalence (Luescher and Pillemer, 1998; Connidis and McMullin, 2002a).

Public and private spheres

Two different meanings of generation exist in everyday culture. One refers to kinship ties and the other to membership of a particular age group, sharing certain social and historical characteristics. The former most commonly relates to the private sphere of family relations – the 'small generational contract' – and the latter to the public sphere of age-based cohorts travelling through time together – the 'big generational contract'. Both are closely intertwined, enjoying considerable overlap as a source of personal identity, like in the more public arenas of policy, work and media debates. As Clain (2005) points out, the social meaning of generation is influenced by socially structured opportunities; values, lifestyles and existential meanings; as well as shared ideological reference points. Intergenerational relationships exist at the interface between private and public spheres (Biggs, 2007). They are *public* as they are subject to social policy and influenced by social perceptions of old age and generational conduct expectations. Intergenerational relationships are *private* in so far as generations are commonly thought of and highlighted within the interpersonal sphere of the family. Moreover, generation in the private sphere of the family denotes age-based locations in families. This implies that the concept of generation as a family term means social relations among members of different ages. As McDaniel (2008) states: 'generation, in this sense, has a fluidity and dynamism that it does not have when it is equated with birth cohort' (p. 3). These distinctions are marked by expectations of care and material transfers that are often explicit. Theoretically, the family has been seen as the principal arena for expressions of intergenerational solidarity as well as rivalry.

Attias-Donfut (2005; 2007), Arber and Attias-Donfut (2000) and Kohli (2007) introduce the perspective of the need to define a generation with regard to both society – the horizontal level context – and to the family (the lineage position) – vertical level context – referring to a feeling of generational belonging and to questions of generational awareness which exist at the intersection of these axes. According to their view, generations are developing all the time not just via specific points in time. The sequence of generations in the family directly conditions the position of the individual in the economic, political and cultural spheres (Biggs and Lowenstein, forthcoming).

Bengtson *et al.* (2005) articulate the linking role of generations to cohorts. In their view, public cultural experience associated with a particular historical cohort could contain a potential for conflict between individuals who belong to a different cohort, with differing cultural and historical expectations both in the public societal sphere and in the private sphere of the family. Generations within the private world of the family hold the potential to smooth out these cultural discontinuities and promote harmonious relations but need an appropriate mechanism, like a high Generational Intelligence as elaborated in Chapter 1.

Families and global ageing

Marshall (forthcoming) argues that if the theoretical perspectives of political economy or critical theory are applied to the phenomenon of global ageing and family the more harmonious picture painted by Bengtson (2001) and Bengtson and Lowenstein (2003) would be quite different. In his view, an ageing person is placed in a family context, but broader contexts related to globalization, which influence family life, should also be considered. He emphasizes three main aspects: first, the growing complexity of intergenerational family relations like greater diversity in intergenerational financial support patterns; second, the need for people to work longer thus delaying the timing of retirement, which will change the nature of family life in the retirement years; and third, the need to increase fertility as otherwise the levels of support families can provide is diminishing. He notes, however, that 'these three factors have the potential to affect family life, albeit in ways that are not entirely clear. There is thus a continuing research agenda in the area of global aging and the family' (p. 17).

Other avenues for innovation in models of variation and change in intergenerational family relationships include exploring whether racial and ethnic groups and members of different social classes differ in the glue that binds generations, spouses or non-marital partners, and siblings, and if so, why.

Equally important, is to understand variability in intergenerational relationships within these groups and how the public and private sphere interconnect. It may mean that families should find new avenues and strategies to renegotiate intergenerational family relations and there is a need to introduce and find new operationalizations of family solidarity in a global context as Bengtson (2001) clearly advocates.

Generational Intelligence and family intergenerational relations

Katz *et al.* (2004) suggest that the typical site for social gerontological discourse on generations in later life is 'relations between older parents and their adult children when the parents are becoming frail' (2004: 394). Such situations need the renegotiation of intergenerational relations and mechanisms to ensure such renegotiations. A specific focus in the private sphere of the individual and the family around generations is reflected in the gerontological writings on ageing families.

We also need to interrogate, in the public sphere, how populations respond to the new culture of productive ageing, how policies fit with everyday experience of intergenerational family relations as part of negotiated balance, for example between work and family life, and what strategies people adopt to increase generational cooperation and reduce conflict and ambivalence.

The phenomenological understanding of Generational Intelligence (Biggs and Lowenstein, forthcoming) would raise some basic issues that have not been at the forefront of debate on generational consciousness in families and societies. Such issues include the expectations, beliefs and resources that each individual brings into the intergenerational familial and societal exchange. Furthermore, exploring how conscious are they of what they bring and how is this performed and negotiated within the encounter. Additionally, the impact it has on process, outcome and potential for connection, conflict or ambivalence between family generations. Finally, what is needed to acquire awareness and building capacity for understanding different generations and their needs.

Understanding the phenomenology of the concept, i.e. how generation is experienced and how a multiplicity of different influences contribute to a singular

experience that people use to navigate their social world, can contribute in bridg-
ing the private sphere of family relations and the public world, for example, of
work. This will be reflected within a life-course perspective linking the individual,
the family and the society along the life-course of different family members. It is
partly embedded in the assumption that generation is experienced in immediate
action as a phenomenological whole, even though it may arise from attitudes to
life-course, family or cohort. As relationship between cooperation, conflict and
ambivalence is currently theoretically contested.

It could be argued that sustainable intergenerational family relationships will
need to rely on increased levels of generational insight, empathy and mutually
negotiated action. Intelligence of this sort facilitates interplay between different
levels of understanding associated with intergenerational exchanges. It would be
especially imperative during times of transitions along the life-course of different
family members, like children growing up and leaving the parental home, retirement or dependency in deep old age.

Generational Intelligence and especially a high Generational Intelligence might
be developed more easily within the framework of generational family relations
based on a life-course approach. Experiences of various family generations along
the life-course, like entering into parenthood and grandparenthood, influence
social pathways and needs renegotiations of roles and behaviours. Thus, developing a high Generational Intelligence should provide avenues to understand such
different experiences. From the intergenerational ambivalence perspective, adult
family generations have to work harder on renegotiating generational relationships if life transitions prove stressful, such as during retirement or making a
decision which of the siblings will assume a caregiving role for older parents.
Here, again acquiring a high Generational Intelligence might be productive to deal
with ambivalence within the family realm. Ward (2008) proposed the concept of
collective ambivalence suggesting that incorporating information from all adult
children in a family yields a more complete view of family relations, especially
mixed and negative relations. It might help us understand processes of developing Generational Intelligence and negotiation of ambivalent relationships within
families if the views and feelings of all family members involved are ironed and
brought up front. An intelligent approach to intergenerational relations would
need to address the issue of how individuals become self-consciously aware of
their generational familial status and how far it influences their experience of and
action towards others in their social world, especially within the family system.
Such a conceptual framework reflects both individual (personal agency – life-
course), familial (family groups – solidarity-conflict, ambivalence) and cohort
(generational conflict, rivalry) levels of analysis and impact of societal changes
on them.

Conflict, Solidarity and Ambivalence can be seen as strategies adopted to
negotiate intergenerational family relations along the life-course. Families would
strive towards solidarity as the affective component in intergenerational family
relations was found to be the most salient compared to conflict or ambivalence
(Lowenstein, 2007). When conflict arises, which could be expressed together with

high solidarity (Silverstein *et al.*, 2010) being generationally aware and under-standing self and others might be important for solving conflicts. Once the high Generational Intelligence is arrived at, family members would learn also to live with ambivalence, especially during times of transitions. Families must always decide how to allocate time and money, and the power of individual family members plays a crucial role in these allocation decisions.

Generational Intelligence, thus, as a new conceptual framework could be a useful mechanism in this regard for successfully negotiating and renegotiating generational relationships and reconciling different forms of conflict in changing social structures. Gen I will allow us to significantly expand current theorizing on solidarity-conflict and ambivalence paradigms. The synergies and adaptations that will arise in the process are bound to provide conceptual stimulus for a more generic model of intergenerational family relations. As outlined in previous chapters, such a process might involve three basic elements: finding the appropriate balance between assimilating information from different family generations and accommodating to perspectives which are not only one's own. The second element concerns the need to recognize that one has to undergo separation from others in the family and then return to them. By returning, the distinctiveness of each of the different family generations can be acknowledged. Finally, with growing older the realization sets in that it is not enough to be immersed in the priorities of my own generation within the family context but as reality is more complex, one needs to be engaged with it to accomplish successful and sustainable intelligent negotiations with all family generations. Such a process will contribute to create a critical space where the complex and diversified intergenerational family relations can be played out, tolerated and understood.

7 Generational Intelligence and caregiving

The family and the state

Summary

Population ageing and increased longevity challenge profoundly the current balance between older and younger generations and between formal and informal systems of care. There is ample evidence, though, about the increasingly important role that family caregivers play around the world and the tension this creates between the autonomy of family members and the responsibility of the state to its citizens. Currently, family members form the backbone of long-term care under a variety of welfare systems.

Caregiving is, therefore, one of the central arenas where generational family relations are pronounced and where continued processes of negotiation take place. It is especially manifested in care for older family members. Thus, the aim of this chapter is to outline how Generational Intelligence (Gen I) is perceived and activated in this area and how a high Gen I can foster successful negotiations for issues involved in family elder care.

The chapter deals with several issues which are imperative in the context of family care for frail elders: the nature of what is caregiving: the ability and willingness of the younger generations to support a growing number of older people; the effect of different national contexts and policies on caregiving behaviours. Discussing emerging new avenues of negotiating intergenerational relationships and exploring how a new conceptual framework of Gen I can be activated to ensure successful negotiations between generations and between family members – those providing care and those receiving care.

We will discuss and analyse what is caregiving and characteristics of primary caregivers for frail old family members, examining the outcomes of such care – negative and positive. Following would be an interrogation of the impact of national contexts and policies on such outcomes. Finally, exploration of the role of Generational Intelligence and its impact on reducing negative outcomes as well as fostering positive ones.

Key points

- caregiving for frail older family members is becoming an 'institutionalized' role along the life course;
- the definition and meaning of caregiving;
- the different family members and family generations involved in care provision;
- discussing the various outcomes of long-term informal care for intergenerational family relations, – positive and negative;
- the impact of formal policies and national context on these outcomes;
- exploring the processes that can foster positive outcomes.

Caregiving as a growing social issue

Introduction

As populations age, the proportion of older people (those 65 years or older) increases and that of children (those under the age of 15 years) decreases. For much of the past, children outnumbered the elderly by a factor of more than six to one. Today, the ratio has declined to about three children per one older person. And within the next few decades, perhaps by 2060, the world's elderly population will begin to exceed the population of children, when each group is expected to account for slightly less than one-fifth of the world population (Chamie, 2010). Thus, with fertility rates decreasing, and the deepening of ageing, the age structure of the population will eventually become a polygon with a shorter base and a larger top (Bengtson and Lowenstein, 2003). Increased longevity also causes a secondary ageing process: a growing number of disabled elderly who may need more care and support. Older dependency rates will rise substantially and increasingly fewer adults will care for a growing number of older persons (WHO, 2002a). To this development one can add the phenomenon of co-ageing, where two generations of children who might be aged 68 or 70 years and some processes of frailty had started and their very old parents who might reach the age of 90 years and more, age together, going through some similar life transitions from independence to dependency and conversely, the grandchildren in these families who are at mid-life who might have to care for both parents and grandparents (Kalmijn and Saraceno, 2008). This, of course, means the need for continued renegotiation of family relations. This process adds burdens to families and states, the two major pillars of support in old age, especially where the state is attempting to reduce its role.

Data in the US, for example, show that, in 2007, about 34 million family caregivers provided care for older family members at any given point in time, and about 52 million people provided care at some time during that year (AARP, 2008). This report reveals that the economic value of the aforementioned caregiving increased to $ 375 billion in 2007, up from $ 350 billion in 2006. Data also show that nearly 70 per cent of women work full-time in the US and most of them assume a variety of caregiving responsibilities (Wisensale, 2008). According to the Eurobarometer data, at the beginning of the 2000s, about 17 per cent of adults in quite a number of the EU countries took care of a frail older adult who was not living with them and another 17 per cent did so for an elderly person living with them (Alber and Kohler, 2004).

The inability or unwillingness of societies to continue to meet the needs of older cohorts as well as the inability or unwillingness of workplaces to relate to needs of working carers, alters the balance between family and societal systems in terms of responsibility for elder care (Lowenstein and Daatland, 2006; Walker, 2000a). Growing old within a global community is resulting in hybrid forms of generational ties within the various global networks and flows, creating new forms of care relations, whilst at the same time undermining existing forms of support (Phillipson, 2003). Thus, as the global political and economic climate seems to suggest less government responsibility to be expected in the future for elder care and increased pressure on families, families are entering into new intergenerational caring relations with regard to intensity and duration, which is historically unprecedented. Family care between adults, and especially in old age, thus turns into a major social issue.

Family solidarity and care, however, may be at risk because of demographic factors (EUROSTAT, 2007) and socio-economic changes such as decline in co-residency between generations (Tomassini *et al.*, 2004). Moreover, the rise in divorce rates and expansion of new and possibly weaker family and household forms (cohabiting couples, single-generation households, one parent families, etc) might affect patterns of care. However, family change is not a uniform process but is mediated by institutional factors like legal reforms and different health care systems, as well as by cultural traditions. All these factors impact forms and modes of caregiving and intergenerational family relationships. One consequence is that some family members providing care may not have had any family or societal role models, necessitating a continued renegotiation of relationships (Biggs and Lowenstein, forthcoming). Moreover, it is important to estimate the availability of adult children for elder care, their lifetime risk in taking on parent care responsibilities and the extent to which other siblings share or replace each other in elder care, as this process demands again renegotiation of intergenerational family and sibling relationships.

While the family continues to carry the major responsibility for elder care in most modern welfare states (e.g. Katz *et al.*, 2004), patterns of intergenerational transfers and support are becoming more complex. Further, the issue is not simply one of demographics. It also requires a re-examination of the cultural and intellectual tools we have available to respond positively to these changes.

What is the meaning of care and main characteristics of caregivers

Considerable debate has surrounded the issue of what constitutes caregiving by adult children to older parent. Walker *et al.* (1995) associate caregiving with the criterion of dependence on another person for any activity essential for daily living, This means providing assistance above and beyond the aid given to physically and psychologically healthy family members. The emphasis is on care tasks with a range of instrumental help from helping with shopping or transportation on a regular basis to providing continuous care for a sick, disabled or elderly person, living on their own or with the caregiver, for the well-being of that individual. Care might involve also providing financial help and emotional support. Others had focused on the age-appropriateness of children's care activities, the extent of such care or the impact on the caregivers (Dearden and Becker, 2004).

The central notion behind the concept of informal care and support is the provision of assistance by the family network during times of crisis and transitions. During such times, fruitful negotiations among family members and understanding the needs of different generations is imperative. However, as frailty sets in the demands are higher and caregiving is becoming an activity undertaken by many middle-aged and older family members without proper preparation. The transition into a caregiving situation can be highly stressful when the conditions requiring care are chronic and progressive, as are the majority of later-life illnesses (Aneshensel *et al.*, 1995). Working as a carer is unpaid and brings little positive status (Millward, 1999). The concepts of care and caring are distinguished by Fine, where he focuses on the dual meaning of caring: 'Caring is both the adjective derived from care, used to describe someone who is kind and gives emotional support to others, and a present participle used to describe the practice of giving care' (2007: 29).

Is family care then a 'labour of love' as proposed by Graham (1983) where the younger generations are able and willing to support frail older family members or is it based on a notion that the state is responsible for elder care and aims to lift the burden of caring from families (Glenn, 2000; Leitner, 2003)? If it is a 'labour of love' then it strengthens the conceptual paradigm of intergenerational family solidarity which is thought to underlie motivations for care (e.g. Bengtson and Roberts, 1991; Bengtson, 1993; Attias-Donfut, 2000; Katz *et al.*, 2010). A study by Grundy and Henretta (2006), comparing data from the UK and the US, for example, show that among mid-life women providing help to one or more adult children increased the probability of also providing care to an elderly parent or parent-in-law, thus confirming the solidarity perspective.

Intergenerational family relations, then, become the ground upon which competing demands are played out. This can occur in terms of spatial relations – where different generations are physically located, how and where they interact and for what purpose. It also takes place over time – like the primacy of certain generational priorities at different life-course phases, reflecting changes in life-course experiences and attributes of all family members involved, when generations are most closely in contact and when their life-course transitions tend not to overlap. Thus, the issue of the 'generational contract' relating to the private sphere of intergenerational family transfers and support becomes important for social integration. Social integration concerns the extent to which individual lives are tied to the lives of others and is to a large extent related to their roles and relationships in families (De Jong Gierveld *et al.*, 2009). Research on family transfers, for example, demonstrates, that transfers are considerable, that they occur mostly in the generational lineage, like for our case providing care to frail old family members (Kohli, 2005; Albertini *et al.*, 2007). This would suggest that successful negotiations between different family generations had occurred.

Typically, elder care in the public sphere is not linked to family policy but discussed under 'health policy'. Such a view disregards complex interdependencies across generations. There is some limited literature, though, that has recognized interdependencies often under such headings as 'sandwich generation' and 'generational squeezes' (Agree *et al.*, 2003; Brody, 1981; Evandrou and Glaser, 2004; Penning, 2002; Rosenthal *et al.*, 1996). In French literature, it surfaces under the term 'pivot generation' on whom family relationships and care turn (Attias-Donfut *et al.*, 2005). The diversity of existing family formats creates uncertainty in intergenerational relations, along with new expectations and has specific effects on life-course role transitions like entering into a caregiver role. The structural organization of the family, given the increased prevalence of families with three, four and even five generations is particularly critical for those caregivers in middle age – the sandwiched caregivers – a phase in life when individuals are likely to play multiple roles (Rubin and White-Means, 2009). Grundy and Henretta (2006) pose the hypothesis of 'competing demands' – mid-life or late-middle aged family members, especially women who face commitments to simultaneous support for their elderly parents and their adult but still partly dependent children; and the hypothesis of 'family solidarity' – those with strong commitments to solidarity who will tend to assist both generations rather than prioritize recipients. In their cross-sectional research comparing Great Britain and the United States, they found broad support for the solidarity hypothesis. Somewhat similar results were found in a cross-national research involving four European countries – Norway, Germany, UK and Spain and Israel where solidarity and support were relatively high even in the Nordic countries (Lowenstein, 2007; Katz *et al.*, 2004; Silverstein *et al.*, in press).

Even in the private environment of closed family relations, though, conflict may arise. For example, in three-generational family configurations, the sandwich or pivot generation has to resolve conflicting expectations from ascendant and descendent generations, especially in the area of financial or instrumental support (e.g. Willson *et al.*, 2003).

Several studies show that the ability of the family to cope with conflicts arising from caregiving responsibilities affect the quality of the care provided, and the quality of relations between caregiver and care receiver (Lieberman and Fisher, 1999; Merrill, 1996). Studies on family relations, caregiving and well-being of family members living in multigenerational households also discuss the issue of family conflict (e.g. Pruchno *et al.,* 1997; Lowenstein and Katz, 2000). These studies show that there are issues of conflict especially around privacy and child-rearing or when care burden is experienced. Moreover, some scholars emphasize conflict in intergenerational relations resulting from care responsibilities and competing demands of different generations, which is also reflected in the 'equity debates' (e.g. Williamson *et al.*, 1999) as well as vulnerability in such relationships (Davey and Szinovacz, 2008; Szinovacz, 2007).

About a decade ago, the perspective of intergenerational ambivalence has re-emerged (Luescher and Pillemer, 1998; Connidis and McMullin 2002a). This view suggests that intergenerational family relationships are inherently structured so as to generate ambivalence, and that people use various strategies in their attempts to reconcile ambivalence. To date, there has been limited empirical work to complement the rich theoretical work in this area, especially as related to caregiving issues (see Fingerman, 2001; Pillemer and Suitor, 2002; Willson *et al.*, 2003).

Luescher and Pillemer suggest that intergenerational ambivalence may be most apparent during status transitions, like when caregiving becomes a specified role. Connidis and McMullin (2002b) used a critical perspective to further the discussion by emphasizing imbalances in power and resources embedded in social relationships. When caregiving for a frail older parent becomes a defined role, power relations between adult siblings and older parents change (Dowd, 1980). Accordingly, Cicirelli (2003) discussed the potential for 'paternalism' to 'subtly increase over the course of a care giving relationship' (2003:18–19). This is reflected for example in issues around 'role reversal' when parents become very frail and almost completely dependent on their children. It is especially pronounced when dementia sets in and the caregiving child is turning into his parents' 'father or mother' (Aneshensel *et al.*, 1995).

Walker *et al.* (1995) relate to the need of understanding that perceptions of caregiving may vary by gender, relationship and personal history. Thus, in care relations the variables of gender, relationship of caregiver to care recipient, types of residence e.g. co-residence, race and ethnicity, socio-economic status and the caregiving context should be considered. It has been again and again demonstrated that there is a hierarchy in caregiving situations – the 'hierarchical compensatory model (Cantor, 1975; 1980) which purported that social relationships formed the basis of preferences for receipt of care – turning first to a spouse and then to adult children' (Szinovacz and Davey, 2008). However, limited evidence was presented to support the model (e.g. Penning, 2002).

Findings reveal that women are still the major providers of care to older family members and because of their rising participation in the labour force, they will be confronted with an increasing problem of combining work and care (e.g. Stoller and Miklowski, 2008; Szinovacz, 2008). In co-residence, more instrumental care is likely to be provided and within more traditional ethnic groups like Afro-Americans in the United States more support and exchange within the family is flowing (Jackson *et al.*, 2005).

The outcomes of providing care for longer duration can result in care burden which can be conceived in terms of the balance between the number of very young and very old family members (dependents) and the number of members of the middle generations (carers). The question is can we view caregiving as an extension of long-established patterns of help and support between family generations. If so, Connidis (2001) showed that shifts in support exchange as parents' age is a key transition with major consequences for parent-child ties. It will therefore be useful to consider the developmental timing of transitions in such relationships and, disengaging from them and factors impacting such relationships.

Most care is provided by spouses and adult children, with the later constituting 41.3 per cent of all informal carers (Wolff and Kasper, 2006). Adult children have been shown to comprise the largest category of membership in elders' social networks (Szinovacz and Davey, 2008). About 22 per cent of caregivers provided between 9–20 hours care per week but 24 per cent provided more than 40 hours care per week (Arno, 2002). It is shown, though, that whilst caregiving is primarily constructed as a family issue, it is perhaps more often an intergenerational issue embedded within families. Both women and men act as caregivers, however, the intensity and length of care differs. Women provide more hours of care, higher levels of care and have less choice in taking on care compared to men. These factors increase a woman's risk for emotional stress and lower quality of life (*Care giving in the US,* National Alliance for Caregiving and AARP Report, 2004). Recently, men had been discovered in the caregiving literature (e.g. Calasanti, 2003; Henz, 2006). This is reflected, for example, in increasing levels of part-time employment among men in the EU (e.g. Roman, 2006). However, much variation is contingent on the women in men's lives: wives caregiving, presence of young children mostly daughters, availability of siblings, especially sisters, which shape the amount and kind of caregiving men provide (Gerstel and Gallagher, 2001). There is some empirical evidence that personal involvement of men in family life and in caregiving has benefited the marital relationship (Halperin, 2007). Adult children's decisions about how to care for older parents may involve even more actors if siblings coordinate this responsibility among themselves and with their parents (Pezzin *et al.*, 2005).

In the EUROFAMCARE project, for example, which collected data from six European countries (Germany, Greece, Italy, Poland, Sweden and the UK) (Lamura *et al.*, 2008), it was found that in the private realm of the family emotional bonds of love and affection constituted the principle motivation for providing care (57 per cent or carers), followed by a 'sense of duty' (15 per cent) and a 'personal sense of obligation' (13 per cent). Results of a recent study exploring motivations for care show again the strength of family solidarity, suggesting that affectual solidarity affected the amount of help provided to older parents in three different countries with different welfare regimes and familial traditions – Norway, Spain and Israel. Another important variable was parental need for care while filial norms – the altruistic perspective – had no effect on the amount of help provided to older parents in any of these countries (Katz *et al.*, 2010). The implications of these data is that inspite of care burden and other socio-demographic factors, successful negotiations among family generations regarding care for older parents can be achieved.

Accordingly, we have to assess the heterogeneity and variability of families within different societal and group structures when providing care to family members, and study the outcomes of such care for intergenerational family relations.

Experiences of caregivers – Outcomes of care

Much of the research on issues of care focused, in the beginning, on questions of stress and burden. This was not surprising given the pressures on families. Family expectations and interactions often change when need for care occurs. Family relationships intensify and generational family interactions may become strained as adult children and grandchildren try to balance needs of dependent elders with those of the whole family (Piercy, 1998; Szinovacz and Davey, 2008). This emphasis, though, resulted in decontextualizing family care, focusing exclusively on a single caregiver, who was the primary caregiver. It meant that looking at the broader family context was neglected, for example at the role of other siblings in families and how decisions were made who will become the primary caregiver and what role will other siblings play (Szinovacz, 2008).

Family structure shapes opportunities for engagement, defining and reinforc-ing both meaningful social roles and those roles that are burdensome. The focus should be on family contexts, and on the heterogeneity among caregivers, among different caring families and how decisions are made within families as to who will be a primary caregiver, who is helping and how this process of negotiations and renegotiations, shapes family intergenerational relationships. The question is also what is the impact of caregiving on family carers? Even today, women provide more personal care than men and report more depression and isola-tion. Additionally, studies suggest enduring effects of caregiving. For example, research showed higher mortality and morbidity among caregivers (Schulz and Martire, 2004; Berkman and Kawachi, 2000), impact on both physical and mental health and increases in stress (e.g. Musil *et al.*, 2003), as well as continued eco-nomic hardships (McDonald *et al.*, forthcoming) which may increase poverty in later life (Brodsky *et al.*, 2002; McDonald*et al.*, 1998; Wakabayashi and Donato, 2006). The two greatest predictors of caregivers' physical and emotional strain were reported health of caregivers and whether they feel they had a choice in tak-ing the responsibilities of care.

Work and family commitments may compete at many phases of the life course, but they come together in potential conflict, in particular in late middle age. Some workers may be at the peak of their careers whereas other workers are then approaching retirement, while at the same time they may have older parents at risk of dependency and children in the process of establishing their own careers and families. Studies consistently present associations between family/work con-flict and the implications of such conflict on performance in the workplace (e.g. Evandrou and Glaser, 2004; Voydanoff, 2005). A wide population, mainly women, are more likely to reduce work hours or relinquish their right to paid work outside the home due to family commitments (e.g. Pavalko and Henderson, 2006). It was also found that work hours reductions and labour force exits were unlikely to be recovered after caregiving responsibilities ended (Spiess and Schneider, 2002).

In the next section, we will look at the policy arena as national policy contexts might affect caregiving behaviours and outcomes. So care strategies for renegoti-ating different policy contexts should be identified.

The policy arena

Families operate in the context of larger social institutions that shape how adult children function in the support systems of their older parents. Indeed, families and state institutions intersect to jointly produce portfolios of care and support for the elderly (Minkler and Estes, 1998). That is, the availability of formal elder-support at the macro-national level is expected to create the opportunity structure that shapes care and support decisions at the micro-family level.

Policy provides an important mechanism through which cultural expectations towards adult ageing and caregiving can be influenced, regarding how mid-life and older adults plan for the future (Sidorenko and Walker, 2004). Such planning is not only shaped by national and local policies, but also by the range and use of services available. Social policy in the context of responsibility for elder care reflects a country's vision as a welfare state, its financial capacity to budget for this purpose and the familial, responsibility-based values concerning care for ageing family members.

At the macro level, welfare state structures can be viewed as varying by the degree of responsibility they claim for dependent members in their populations (see Esping-Andersen, 1990; 1999). Different variations exist on the axis between minimum state interventions. In Anglo-Saxon countries such as the US, Australia and England, which have adopted economically liberal regimes, such regimes provide means tested benefits at a low level. On the other hand, in countries like Germany, Denmark and Sweden, which have social democratic regimes, the state guarantees universal benefits and services at high levels, combined with state and family cooperation in caring for family members in need (Esping-Andersen, 1999; Neal and Hammer, 2007). In countries with liberal regimes, a caregiving employee, for example, is expected to rely on personal resources to care for family members, whereas in social democratic countries, the responsibility to meet the needs of employees and their families is perceived to be both private (of the family) and public (of the state) (Den Dulk, 2005). These labels are efficient descriptors, since they conform to known structural orientations of nations towards dependent populations as manifested by service and benefit eligibility and generosity.

Welfare states share a common concern about how to build supportive relationships between families and the state. In so doing, they will inevitably be dealing with questions such as: the balance between families and services systems and what are the relationships between families and services. In other words, how the responsibilities for elder care should be divided between the family, the welfare state and others. Hardly a new theme, but with renewed relevance from the present pressures of population ageing in a climate that constrains welfare state spending. The issue is to understand if access to welfare state services will affect family help negatively – crowding-out or positively – crowding-in.

An example is the Scandinavian countries which developed generous welfare policies (Esping-Andersen, 1999) that reduced dependency upon the family and the normative control of these dependencies. Such an approach is also distinguished by what Esping-Andersen (1999) postulates as 'A de-familializing regime, one which seeks to unburden the household and diminish individuals' welfare dependence on kinship' (1999: 51). A different approach is inherent in the *complementarity approach* which postulates that informal and formal care networks complement each other, each having certain kinds of caregiving responsibilities and capabilities that are best tailored to each particular network structure and can work in partnership (Litwak, 1985). The use of state services strengthens intergenerational relations, not only on a practical level, but also at a symbolic social level, reinforcing a caring society. It also corresponds somewhat to what Esping-Andersen distinguishes as a 'familialistic "one" in which public policy assumes – indeed insists – that households must carry the principal responsibility for their members' welfare' (1999: 51). Formal care is mobilized when crucial elements of the informal network are lacking or when there is a substantial need to assist these networks. This means that families are allowed to choose to care – which is the way in which successful negotiated Generational Intelligence type solutions should be heading, providing an example of a space that can facilitate Generational Intelligence.

There is rich data which show that services complement family care. Data show that welfare support and transfers do not 'crowd out' support from within the family but rather an element of 'crowding in' was evident (Hoff and Tesch-Roemer, 2007). Moreover, some researchers argue for an even stronger case of complementarity, suggesting that a generous welfare state is a stimulant to family solidarity and exchange (Kunemund and Rein, 1999; Lowenstein and Daatland, 2006). This view provides space for generations to interact equally, leaving the tasks to professionals. Clare Wenger's research showed that given the choice both professionals and family carers preferred neutral professional care – so that they could get on with having a normal relationship.

Data from the OASIS project, for example, show that more generous welfare state services have not crowded out the family but have contributed to a change in how families relate, and have helped the generations involved in caregiving to establish more independent relationships. The findings also suggest that family solidarity is not easily lost, considering the fundamental and often existential character of such relationships (Daatland and Lowenstein, 2005). It means the subjective evaluation of being 'well-embedded' in the lives and intimate thinking of people who are important in one's life. Social integration, thus, concerns the extent to which individual lives are tied to the lives of others and is to a large extent related to their roles and relationships in marriage and parenthood. Contacts and exchange of support with the family fall in the heart of the theoretical notions of social embedment and attachment (Attias-Donfut *et al.*, 2005).

People's roles evolve with increasing age (Shaw *et al.*, 2007). After retirement, most contacts with former colleagues fade away, and contacts with members of the community often lessen when children leave the parental home. Moreover, widows generally report a decline in relationships with acquaintances and friends. Several authors address the process that with increasing age, bonds with non-kin will decrease in importance, while the bonds with children and close family members might increase in importance (Carstensen, 1995). The bonds with spouse and children seem to be based on a continued recognition of family obligations as the guidelines for action and part of the cement that keep families together (Daatland and Herlofson, 2003).

The positive value attached by many mid-life carers to family caregiving (Lamura *et al.*, 2008) is probably a critical element in ensuring good quality care for dependent elderly. However, family caregivers need support from integrated formal care services both to aid in the provision of care to older people as well as for the protection of the family caregivers' own health and well-being. Complementing family care, the provision of service support for family caregivers is, therefore, essential and should be part of active public policies.

Thus, it seems that an effective way in which a pluralistic system of care can enhance the ability of the family to meet family care needs is for formal providers to work in partnership with families and with various caregivers within families – a model of shared care. Actually, partnership arrangements between public, private and voluntary agencies are limited but it is an area ripe for development (Walker, 2000a).

Generational Intelligence and caregiving

In light of demographic, social and economic changes, including longer life expectancy, marriage and childbirth at a later stage of life and increased entry rates of women (the traditional family caregivers) into the labour market, society is faced with new challenges. These challenges include assisting families to continue supporting their ageing members and helping in renegotiating family relationships related to caregiving. The perception in the literature of caregiving relationships has gradually shifted from the long-standing approach that tended to focus on the adult children's perspective and emphasized adverse outcomes for both caregiver and care recipient, to a view that takes into account a more dynamic and interactive relationship between adult children and older parents. Growing old within a global community is resulting in hybrid forms of generational ties within various global networks, creating new forms of care relations and at the same time undermining existing forms of support (Phillipson, 2003).

While the family continues to carry the major responsibility for elder care in most modern welfare states (Katz *et al.*, 2003; Lowenstein, 2007), patterns of intergenerational solidarity and support are becoming more complex. Thus, one of the challenges is to maintain the intergenerational contract (Rossi and Rossi, 1990). The intergenerational contract is based on the notion that each generation invests in the human capital of the next and is taken care of at the end of its life by the generations in which it has invested. Hence, each generation cares twice (once for the previous generation and once for the next generation) and is taken care of twice (as a child and in old age). Within a family context, women are the traditional brokers of the intergenerational contract, providing most of the informal care to children and aged older parents and other aged relatives.

More generations within intergenerational families are living alongside each other for longer time periods, where the 'sandwich' or 'pivot' generation (family members supporting their parents and children at the same time) has expanded to include not only young people caring for elderly parents and young children, but also people in middle age, who are caring for parents, adult offspring and even grandchildren. A large segment of this population is in the workforce, and society is facing the need to support and help them cope with the (often conflicting) roles of work and elder care.

Primary caregivers, though, have then to understand and be aware of the 'age other' – the care receiver – as well as other actors in the family systems like siblings and/or grandchildren. Moreover, they have to learn to renegotiate so that all involved would understand and relate to the various needs of caregivers and care receivers. The care receiver and other family members, on the other hand, have also to be critically aware of the 'age other' – the caregiver. However, as more women, who are still the traditional caregivers, are entering the workforce and with changing demographics and changing roles and expectations, it is important to re-focus attention to the processes that underpin these kinds of relationship. This suggests an even stronger need to go through the process and steps which will ensure acquiring a high Generational Intelligence.

Acquiring such high Generational Intelligence will mean understanding of two key aspects of intergenerational relations. First, the degree to which it is possible to place oneself in the position of the age-other, either a caregiver or a care receiver, and second, the possibility of working towards negotiated and sustainable solutions between the different generations in the family who are involved like other siblings or grandchildren. One has to understand that a critical distance has to be created and thus, becoming first consciously aware of one's own generational identity. Such a process means that it is necessary to separate and then return to the 'age other', so that the distinctiveness of each position would be recognized. It will involve also becoming critically aware of the values and attitudes underpinning beliefs about intergenerational relations, filial norms and obligations to provide care. This will provide an avenue for action to achieve successful and sustainable negotiations which will facilitate one's ability to fulfil the caregiver role successfully. As Marshall *et al.* argue, the nature of caregiving relations 'rests on a delicate balance between reciprocity, affection and duty' (1987: 407). For example, it has been demonstrated that reciprocity is an important element in older parent–adult-child relations (e.g. Lowenstein *et al.*, 2008) and it features significantly in the ideological construction of the caring relationships (e.g. Qureshi and Walker, 1989). In terms of Generational Intelligence, it means sometimes perceiving the needs of the 'age-other' – the care receiver as well as one's own children and sometimes grandchildren – as priority to one's own needs. It should be considered, though, alongside emotional relationships which were developed along the life course (Roberts *et al.*, 1991; Lowenstein, 2007) and societal norms and beliefs (Finch and Mason, 1993). Given the diversity of family ties, though, it might be differently negotiated within different family contexts and in varying family cultures.

8 Generational Intelligence and elder mistreatment

Summary

Elder abuse and neglect is an extreme example of what can go wrong in caring relationships. It is not exclusively intergenerational in form, but is distinctive in so far as it is defined as a problem of old age and that carers other than spouses are more often than not younger than the nominated victim. Mistreatment has most commonly been identified in families and in institutional care, both of which are intergenerational contexts. It exists in the context of ageist stereotyping that may act as permessors for such behaviour. In this chapter, we look at the way that mistreatment has been defined and has emerged as a social problem. It is suggested that the area has spread in terms of awareness-raising, but has not grown in terms of understanding of the issues involved. The field has been subject to binary oppositions that may indicate the need for higher degrees of Generational Intelligence to be at work. In order to cope with the complexity of damaged intergenerational relations, the adult-adult nature of the relationship needs to be recognized and a sufficient degree of ambiguity and ambivalence tolerated so that the problem can be contained and understood.

Key points

- Elder mistreatment (abuse and neglect) is an age-specific form of failed relationship that is often intergenerational in character.
- It exists in the context of ageist stereotypes, and has been defined as a form of interpersonal behaviour.
- The area has spread as an international concern, but has not developed significantly in terms of understanding the phenomenon.
- A generationally intelligent response to the problem could involve recognizing of complexity and a move away from binary oppositions.
- Accepting that mistreatment exists in the context of adult-adult relationships requires considerable tolerance of ambivalent feelings, that facilitate negotiated intergenerational solutions.

Introduction

Elder mistreatment, the abuse or neglect of older adults, is perhaps one of the most extreme instances in which generational antagonisms come to the surface in contemporary societies. There are a growing number of national prevalence studies, from North America, Europe, Australasia and parts of East Asia, that indicate that between 180 and 20 older people per thousand are likely to be victims of abuse depending upon culture and measures used. Almost all of these studies have taken place amongst people living in community settings and may therefore exclude the most vulnerable elders who may be suffering from dementia or living in residential or nursing homes. Since its foundation in 1997, the International Network for the Prevention of Elder Abuse (INPEA) has grown significantly, with a spreading regional and national membership. On June 15, 2006 the first World Elder Abuse Awareness Day, which has now become an annual event, was launched at the United Nations in New York. Awareness of the mistreatment of older citizens is therefore increasing as both a global and local phenomenon.

However, while awareness of abuse and neglect may be spreading, it would be difficult to argue that understanding of the problem has grown significantly from the initial studies that took place in the United States in the late 1960s and 1970s, as reviewed in Pillemer and Wolf's (1986) 'Elder Abuse: Conflict in the Family'. Much of the literature in this area continues to consist of small case studies or reports on particular service initiatives. Conceptual development has tended to rely on importing ideas from other areas, such as child abuse, domestic or intimate partner violence (Biggs, 1993).

Elder mistreatment also sits at the crossroads of scientific research, policy development and professional concern. And it is perhaps in the nature of vulnerability in later life, that there has not been a strong voice from the nominated victims of mistreatment. There is therefore a vacuum at the centre of debate, which has to be filled with some form of empathic understanding or it will serve as a space in which responses to vulnerable old age are acted out. Each of these factors has lead to a continuing debate about the definition and scope of the problem. It appears that researchers, policy-makers and concerned others, keep returning to and worrying about this aspect of the problem, while each new iteration of a definition makes comparisons between different studies and initiatives more difficult, as it is less easy to compare like with like.

A strange element of the debate on elder mistreatment is that after almost 50 years of awareness of the phenomenon, mistreatment is still commonly thought to be a new social problem. And, as Richard Bonnie, Chair of the US National Research Council review of elder mistreatment pointed out very little progress has been made in its understanding: 'In 1986 a consensus conference was convened . . . the conclusions and recommendations reached are strikingly similar to those appearing in this report' (Bonnie and Wallace, 2003: 23).

It is as if abuse and neglect act as a reflection of public unwillingness to encounter intergenerational relationships when they go bad. They are not, in some profound way, within empathic range in the same way as the safeguarding of childhood or of intimate partner relationships might be. And while it is important to distinguish between forms of mistreatment and a systemic susceptibility to ageism, ageism in the evasive sense of withdrawing from unpleasant personal and systemic 'futures', may act as a block against progress in understanding extreme negative forms of interpersonal intergenerational behaviour.

These tensions, when put together, raise questions about what is meant by understanding an emotionally charged issue such as elder mistreatment. What, from the position of a critical generational perspective, and one that attempts to examine what is going on in terms of Generational Intelligence, are we trying to understand? One response to this question would hinge on the relationship between personal, interpersonal and social influences on behaviour. The latter forms a ground upon which more personal beliefs and behaviours are played out and arise as issues with different levels of depth of understanding. It would be part of a psychosocial approach that, as Stenner and Taylor (2008) argue, yields a politics which attends to the subjective and emotional experiences of welfare users and providers alongside issues of justice. In other words, and in the broadest sense, the study of elder mistreatment interacts with emotional dynamics arising from the phenomenon, which include attitudes and expectations between generations and leads some element of inquiry to be dominant and others to be suppressed, some immersive and some open to reflective understanding.

Ways of thinking about social issues

At one level, usually manifest in policy development, responses to mistreatment can be seen as part of a 'social problem approach'. A new phenomenon has arrived that needs a response. Understanding of the issue goes through certain phases of recognition and reaction and is eventually found a socially constructed place in which it can be 'made sense of' (Blumer, 1971; Schneider, 1985). This then becomes the taken as given and largely unreflective 'common-sense' view of the problem within any given context, which determines the nature of the response and the distribution of resources, their direction and priority. Mistreatment may, for example, be seen as a welfare issue or a criminal justice issue, a problem of care or of crime. And depending upon that position, public understanding of the problem and institutional responses cohere around a particular set of social relations and expectations. In terms of abuse, the use of terms such as victim and perpetrator would push the problem towards criminal justice, while the association of abuse with situations involving family members and care homes pushes it towards welfare-based explanations and actions. As it sits at a boundary between different forms of institutional response, as defined by the culturally contingent and historically dependent evolution of the institutions themselves, mistreatment becomes contested territory and within this understanding of social problems, varies in its meaning and perceived importance. Policy debates then often take the form of how to coordinate responding between different institutional blocs, such as social work, the police and medicine. A disadvantage of the social problems approach is that a problem is perceived as very much as existing 'in itself'. While its scope and nature may be subject to fierce debate, the emergence of the problem does not threaten the goodness of society in general, and relations between generations in particular. Rather, the discovery of the problem reinforces an overall sense of a good society that responds humanely to the difficult situations its citizens may face. Resources are used to ameliorate or eradicate the discrete problem, to bring it back under control. It permits forms of legitimate rescue. The problem itself is framed in terms of vulnerability and risk with respect to a limited set of negative behaviours. From this perspective, the emphasis is, at root, on finding ways of responding to discrete acts of mistreatment.

At a deeper level, understanding of the problem uses could be referred to as the 'mirror' critique. This is perhaps best captured in the words of the existential philosopher and social critic, De Beauvoir, although it is also reflected in the work of Foucault (1977). According to De Beauvoir's famous statement: 'By the way in which society behaves toward its old people it uncovers the naked, and often carefully hidden truth about its real principles and aims' (1970: 35).

This position differs radically from the first approach in so far as it would not see phenomena such as abuse as isolated problems or system aberrations. Rather, they disclose something fundamental about the nature of contemporary societies. As such, social problems like elder mistreatment cannot be 'fixed' without addressing core building blocks in the distribution of power between groups in society, in this case defined primarily by age and generation. Events that appear to be on the periphery of society, that are marginal to its main concerns, are, according to this view, more likely to reflect its underlying structure. This is in part because on the periphery, they are less subject to routine self-censorship or scrutiny, even though they may be more prone to 'policing'. Marginal events hold a mirror to society. They also have liminal qualities that afford a glimpse into an alternative to official versions and assumptive realities that hold every-day expectations in place. Mistreatment, which itself often occurs in transitional or contested situations, challenges idealized versions of intergenerational or peer relations, and in so doing, reintroduces notions of conflict, rivalry and age prejudice.

According to Foucault (1977), the emergence of a new social problem provokes a 'swarming' of professions around it that both defines the problem and shapes the professions in question. An interaction between the collection of knowledge about the phenomenon and the power that knowledge lends to shape the way further information is collected, legitimizes a particular understanding and particular power relationships. New problems, such as elder abuse, are not simply discovered and responded to by existing authorities, rather legitimized professional activities emerge at the same time as the problem itself evolves and becomes visible. This idea is similar to Estes' critique of 'the ageing enterprise' (1979; 1993) in which professional and commercial interests attempt to define old age in certain ways, largely to commodify it. The two perspectives differ in so far as Estes primarily sees ageing as subjected to political and economic exploitation, whereas Foucault would argue that power relations are implicit within the detail of everyday rela-tionships. Both link us to the way in which we make sense of unexpected and disturbing circumstances that do not simply reflect individual circumstances, but reflect deep-seated predispositions within social life.

In terms of Generational Intelligence, mistreatment would provoke a contest between emotionally simplified solutions that split actors and actions into opposites, such as good-bad, active-passive, victim-perpetrator, and a challenge to engage with emotionally and conceptually difficult material. It would require a more nuanced understanding of the interactions between personal, interpersonal and systemic factors in the creation of a phenomenology of mistreatment. It would not stop at calling 'something must be done' and a jump into over-hasty action, but would go on to examine how sustained and negotiated solutions might emerge.

Public assumptions and research evidence

A starting point would be to examine the immersive or common-sensual understanding of elder mistreatment and compare this to available research evidence.

Stones and Pittman asked a group of Canadian women and men with an average age of 38 years, and from a spread of occupations, about their attitudes to abuse and neglect. They found wide variation in attitudes, but that views on mistreatment varied most strongly according to general social attitudes and underlying belief structures held by respondents rather than issues specific to the problem at hand: 'Attitude moderation is associated with complex but coherent beliefs, whereas extremity is associated with simpler or conflicting belief structure' (1995: 69). McCreadie and Biggs (2006) found that focus group participants aged 65 years and older, tended to reproduce a series of common-sensual myths about elder abuse. Childs *et al.* (2000) US study of students and people in mid-life, found that female midlifers were more likely to judge mistreatment more harshly than other groups. In each study, attitudes to mistreatment varied according to a number of factors unrelated to the information supplied about the problem itself.

Hussein *et al.* (2007) analysed a BBC survey of 1,000 adults' awareness of 'elder abuse'. They found that older people believed there was less mistreatment than younger people, women believed there was more than men and that there were regional variations in these perceptions. Overall, respondents estimated that 11.4 per cent of older adults suffered from physical abuse, 4.9 per cent from stealing (financial), 0.8 per cent from sexual abuse and 20.7 per cent from humiliation (psychological). In 2008, a Eurobarometer study undertaken by the European Commission found that 47 per cent of European citizens thought that 'poor treatment, abuse and neglect' was widespread, with considerable variation between the 27 member states. Romania reached the highest with 86 per cent and Cyprus the lowest at 17 per cent, with the UK (47 per cent), France (43 per cent) and Germany (42 per cent) in the middle. When asked what level of risk there was for older dependent citizens, abuse of property reached 67 per cent, psychological abuse 64 per cent, physical 52 per cent and sexual 31 per cent.

These common sense assumptions about mistreatment do not fit well with research evidence. In fact, they are a significant over-estimate. The closest prevalence figures currently available are from the UK community survey of older adults (O'Keefe *et al.*, 2007; Biggs *et al.*, 2009), that found a figure of 2.6 per cent for abuse and neglect by family, friends and caregivers, extending to 4 per cent once neighbours and acquaintances were taken into account. The most common form of mistreatment was neglect at 1.1 per cent, financial abuse at 0.7 per cent, psychological and physical, both at 0.4 per cent and sexual harassment at 0.2 per cent. Even the most prevalent comparable study (Lowenstein *et al.*, 2009) estimated mistreatment to reach 18 per cent. German estimates reached 1.45 per cent (Goergen, 2007), and Spanish estimates between 0.5 per cent and 4.5 per cent depending upon whether nominated victims or carers were asked (Iborra, 2008).

When these assumed and actual figures are compared, it is clear that not only is there wide variation in the public mind, it can also vary from the research evidence. In general, public estimates are significantly higher than research figures and occasionally identify a different order of risk.

Development of a concept over time

When Foucault (1976/1981) discussed the development of knowledge about an emerging social phenomenon, he identified two trends which can take place. First, there is an attempt to increasingly specify, via ever more precise classification, the fine detail of a newly identified domain. Second, there is a tendency to channel the phenomenon into particular visible forms, to make it public and manageable. One way, he suggested of examining these processes at work would be to study the genealogy of the issue, the development of a concept over time in order to see which processes become dominant and which are dropped by the wayside (Visker, 1995). It may be possible, then, to examine the definitional domain of elder mistreatment to critically assess the development of this social problem.

The spread of mistreatment

The worldwide awareness of elder mistreatment, associated with the International Network for the Prevention of Elder Abuse – INPEA, and the inauguration of a United Nations awareness day is a considerable achievement. As interest in the issue has expanded, interest in the definition of the problem has also become a core focus of discourse. The refinement of definitions has taken two routes. First, there has been an attempt to achieve a universally acceptable form of words that encapsulates the problem. Second, successive studies have examined the types of abuse and neglect that might be covered, resulting in lists of abusive or neglectful behaviours, plus types of victims and perpetrators. Thus, any genealogy of mistreatment needs to examine the development of universalizing definitions and of typological definitions. In fact, even the use of the phrase 'mistreatment' is itself the product of successive refinement and re-interpretation.

Initial attempts to specify mistreatment tended to be simple statements, which can now be seen as amalgams that were later to evolve into general and typological forms. Eastman, in the UK refers to 'the systematic maltreatment, physical, emotional or financial of an elderly person by a care-giving relative' (1984:

23) and was cited with approval by the British Department of Health (1993). In the US, Johnson referred to 'Self or other inflicted suffering unnecessary to the maintenance of the quality of life of the older person' (1986: 101). This definition was adopted by Pillemer and Wolf in their seminal work (1986: 89). At about this time Pillemer and Finkelhor (1988), in the first recorded prevalence study, indicated that in addition to perpetration by adult-child on parents; which had been the dominant focus of Congressman Claude Pepper's hearings on abuse in the late 1970s (National Research Council, 2003); spousal abuse was a significant element. Both were placed in the context of family caregiving, while the hearings highlighted caregiver stress as an important factor, and the spousal element focused on parallels with domestic violence.

Universal definitions

In 1991, Hudson, used a 'Delphi' method to obtain a cross section of expert researcher and professional opinion on the scope of the problem, generating both a taxonomy and definitions. Mistreatment was described as:

> Destructive behaviour that is directed toward an older adult, occurs within the context of a relationship connoting trust and is of sufficient intensity and/or frequency to produce harmful physical, psychological, social and/or financial effects of unnecessary suffering, injury, pain, loss and/or violation of human rights and poorer quality of life for the older adult.
>
> (Hudson, 1991: 14)

As awareness of mistreatment spread, a running problem within the definitional discourse had been how to identify, and label different protagonists and resolve the question of the relationship between parties. Some way had to be found that could include a diverse set of context-dependent relations, such as children, partners, paid helpers, workers and residents in institutions, plus advice and interventions by a number of professionals, which nevertheless extended across different locations of abuse such as domestic environments, hospitals or residential care.

In 1994, the UK-based charity, Action on Elder Abuse (2010) (AEA) undertook its own Delphic consultation, which came up with the following definition: 'Elder Abuse is a single or repeated act, or lack of appropriate action, occurring within any relationship where there is an expectation of trust, which causes harm or distress to an older person' (p. 1).

And while alternative generic definitions have been proposed since, such as by Eagle (1994), and Podniek's (2007) environmental scan, examined later; the AEA statement has since been adopted by the World Health Organization (2002a) and cited by the European Commission (2008).

A key ingredient that both Hudson and AEA include is the notion of a 'position of trust' which has since been expanded by the US National Research Council Panel (Bonnie and Wallace, 2003). 'A Trust relationship', they claim, includes:

A caregiving relationship or other familial, social or professional relationship where a person bears or has assumed responsibility for protecting the interests of the older person or where expectations of care or protection arise by law or social convention . . . The category of relevant relationships includes not only caregivers, but also to other family members or even unrelated people (e.g., lawyers) who are aware of the elder's vulnerability and exploit it. The panel uses the phrase 'trust relationships' to denote the relevant relationships.

(Boonie, and Wallace, 2003: 41–42)

The notion of 'trust relationship' is useful in so far as it unpeels notions of obligation and care from particular settings. Focusing on trust relationships rather than particular role relations appeared to add flexibility so that definitions of abuse and neglect could be extended beyond their original locations. It expands the scope of who might be in an abusive relationship. However, it also introduces a lack of specificity in terms of who is expecting trust and whether the undertaking is necessarily reciprocal, relational and justifiable.

In Eagle's (1994) definition, 'elder abuse is any form of conduct toward, or neglect of an elderly person, treated as such, who is or maybe adversely affected thereby' and a more recent 'Worldview Environmental Scan' (Podnieks, 2007) defined elder abuse as

Any harm done to an older person that undermines that person's physical, emotional, spiritual or social well being. The forms of abuse can include, but are not limited to, physical, sexual, and emotional abuse, financial exploitation, neglect, intimidation, coercion, discrimination, and self-neglect.

(Eagle, 1994: 1)

The characteristic feature of both of these statements is that they use, even more liberally than the AEA position, inclusive terms such as 'any', 'is or maybe', 'include and are not limited to'. This significantly increases the spread and scope of what might be considered mistreatment, but leave few clues as to how to compare, test for and respond to different forms of elder mistreatment.

Typologies

As generic, universalizing definitions moved towards ever widening meanings of what might be classified as abusive behaviour, the number of types also increased. Pillemer and Finkelhor's (1988) original Boston study, referred to physical violence, chronic verbal aggression and neglect, with neglect being added because it fell under the same category in the state legislature. Since then, forms of mistreatment have grown such that now mistreatment is generally accepted to include physical, psychological, financial and sexual forms, in addition to neglect and a critical focus on discourses based on human rights and dignity (Bonnie and Wallace, 2003; Tinker *et al.*, 2010; Biggs and Stevens, 2010, Lowenstein and Doron, 2008). To these have been added: structural and societal abuse, neglect and abandonment, disrespect and ageist attitudes, and legal and financial abuse (WHO, 2002b; 2008); with self-neglect being added by the US National Center for Elder Abuse (2009). Other phrases such as emotional abuse and discriminatory abuse can also be found (Department of Health, 2000; 2008). The Environmental scan (Podnieks, 2007) expands the typological horizon ever further to include physical, sexual and emotional abuse, financial exploitation, neglect, intimidation, coercion, discrimination, self-neglect, leaving space for other forms not yet thought of.

Prevalence

During this time, estimates of prevalence also grew at an incremental rate. Prevalence refers to the number of cases of a given phenomenon would be expected to occur within any one population and is expressed as a percentage. There are now at least eight prevalence studies reported in the scientific literature, including two from the US, two from Canada, one from Hong Kong, one from Israel and four from Europe. Four of these have been based on the family, five on community samples and one on the criminal justice system. The time periods covered by different reports vary according to definition and include: 'since 60 years', 'since 65 years' and 'for the past 5 years' plus one year, and finally, three months. The type of abuse has also varied depending on the study in question.

Despite wide methodological and contextual differences, comparison of the single overall prevalence figures arising from each study is often taken to show an increase in mistreatment. Until studies, published between 2007 and 2008 from Germany, Spain and the UK, the trajectory for prevalence had been taken to be increasing, with estimates rising from 2.6 per cent in the original Boston study of 1986, to 4 per cent from Canada, 5.6 per cent from Holland, 22 per cent from Hong Kong and in 2006, 18.4 per cent from Israel (HRSDC, 2009). Other studies did not offer an overall prevalence rate. The counter-intuitive fall in prevalence in more recent studies produced disquiet within what might be called the 'elder mistreatment enterprise' (Action on Elder Abuse, 2008).

Spreading, not growing

Taken together, trends in the literature on generic definitions, typologies and even certain prevalence studies, indicate a spreading of the territory covered by mistreatment to include ever broadening horizons. This spreading territory, combined with increased detail, is typical of Foucault's 'swarming' effect: a process of simultaneously universalizing and a specifying. However, while more items have been added to the surfaces of mistreatment, few of these studies offer a greater understanding of the dynamics that maintain or differentiate specific forms as they are identified. It is in this sense that the area has spread, but has not grown.

Current work on mistreatment, then, leaves significant gaps in its understanding, while permitting ever broader forms of activity to be included within its remit. A genealogical approach, even a preliminary one such as outlined earlier, indicates important developmental trends, but rather than highlighting which influences come in and out of focus over time, it has been more instructive as identifying an almost wilfully simple additive process. It is not, then that mistreatment suffers from 'definitional disarray' (Pillemer and Finkelhor, 1988) so much as a progressive pattern of expansion. Few items have been lost, but surprisingly, few new perspectives have come into play. If there have been lost issues, it may be more accurate to describe them as areas that have been persistently underdeveloped, including a willingness to critically assess the relationship between changing political boundaries and their effects upon how the problem has been perceived, the motivations and complexity of adult-adult relationships, the dynamics of intergenerational relationships and the influence of a somewhat specialized, but nevertheless effective ageing enterprise.

How is it that the dynamics of interpersonal relations has been underemphasized, when this has not been the case in cognate areas such as child abuse and domestic violence (McCluskey and Hooper, 2000)? Generationally intelligent curiosity is raised by this genealogy, in part, because it is unclear why the study of forms of mistreatment specifically concerning elders are so lacking in sophistication.

Boundaries, trust and adult-adult relations

For elder abuse to make sense, definitions must set boundaries around what can be included, otherwise the phenomenon loses meaning. The NRC panel recognized this, and have worked hard to exclude self-neglect and classify mistreatment as an interpersonal issue. 'Mistreatment' it is argued 'conveys two ideas; that some injury, deprivation, or dangerous condition has occurred to the elder person and that someone else bears responsibility for causing the condition or failing to prevent it' (National Research Council, 2003: 40).

Abuse and exploitation by strangers is also excluded as these do not imply an ongoing 'trust relationship'. The panel also recognized that abuse and neglect have different dynamics and should be treated as separate phenomena. A serious problem, in the US context lies in the diversity of state legislature (Daly and Jogerst, 2006) and prompted a need to develop 'objective, uniform research definitions that are disentangled from statutory variation and from contingent or subjective value judgements'. (National Research Council, 2003: 34).

As policy definitions, at least in the UK, have tended to use service eligibility as a criterion for including cases as mistreatment (Department of Health, 2000), and that these change over time independently of need, a scientific mistrust of policy is probably justified on both sides of the Atlantic.

Related areas, such as adult bullying, which Salin defines as 'repeated and persistent negative acts towards one or more individuals which involve a perceived power imbalance and create a hostile . . . environment' (2003: 1214–15) are clearly restricted to refer to 'affective relationship conflict' that is 'interpersonal in nature'. Similarly Brammer refers to domestic, or intimate partner, violence as: 'persons who have had an intimate personal relationship with each other which is or was of significant duration' (2006: 50).

In each case, creating clear boundaries is seen as an aid to locating a social problem and distinguishing it from related phenomena, or broader social issues.

Putting boundaries around the problem is particularly important with respect to issues that invite intuitive and emotional reactions. As has been shown, trust relations and the associated presumption of responsibility for another person have become a key, if problematic, component of attempts to clarify the meaning of mistreatment. Bauman (1995), it will be recalled, has argued that responsibility for the other, a core element of trust relations, is 'shot through with ambivalence' (1995: 2).

From a gerontologically intelligent position, where clear boundaries and recognizing connections are important, trust relations tacitly draw attention to long-standing but neglected aspects of elder mistreatment. The first of these is that, in contrast to child mistreatment, elder mistreatment is an adult-adult interaction. In other words, it assumes that both parties are capable of making decisions about the nature of the relationship itself. This point is reinforced by the observation that, with minimal exception (Cooper *et al.*, 2009), existing prevalence studies have excluded persons with dementia, and assume that respondents are capable of independent judgement. In the case of families, there is persuasive evidence that care relations are negotiated, and do not work on the basis of externally imposed obligation (Finch, 1995; Lowenstein *et al.*, 2007). An implication is that mistreatment would need to be seen as a longitudinal phenomenon within relationships, that it exists in the context of relations that are subject to debate, even when these appear have broken down, and an understanding of the phenomenon would need to take into account the views of each party even when it may be externally defined as abusive.

While one would be forgiven for thinking that discussion of mistreatment has been assumed to be 'hidden' (Action on Elder Abuse, 2004) or 'missing' (WHO, 2002b), there is evidence that protagonists are willing to talk openly about it. Juklestad (2001), for example found that paid carers were willing to discuss abuse, including personal involvement, in a problem-solving manner. Iborra's (2008) study found that proportionally more abuse was reported by family caregivers than by older adults themselves. The only current prevalence study of care home abuse (Pillemer and Moore, 1989) relied heavily on careworker's self report. The negotiative nature of mistreatment is also suggested by work that shows that different cultures tolerate different levels of dispute and conflict within families (Lowenstein *et al.*, 2006). There is also a parallel literature on the abusive behaviour of older adults towards care-givers, which is rarely drawn upon within mistreatment discourse. Jackson (1996) has edited a volume that included instances of sexual harassment, dogmatism and manipulative behaviour from older adults, while Banerjee *et al.* (2008) document a growing problem of violence against support workers in long-term care.

The point here is not to minimize the pain and hurt that mistreatment can cause, but to recognize that there are counter-intuitive trends that have largely been eclipsed in the dominant discourse. These militate for an adult to adult and two-way intergenerational understanding of the problem and its solution. Not to do so would seem to replicate an infantilization and reinforcement of a passive role for older adults. Trust, then, needs to be seen as a reciprocal relationship, involving negotiation and the recognition of complex emotions including pain, guilt and reparation.

Simplifying oppositions

The most commonly found simplifying mechanism in the literature on mistreatment is that of identifying victims and perpetrators, which if used as a binary and mutually exclusive opposition, lends strength to an immersive approach to the problem. It is, however, the standard way of discriminating between populations in prevalence studies because it lends itself to the identification of discrete parties that are locatable and measurable. It is also closely tied to a legalistic understanding of how the problem should be addressed, fixing protagonists at one or other pole. Contrary to the trends set up by recognizing the adult-adult nature of abusive relationships, it segregates individuals into active and passive parties, clarifies the third role of rescuer and gives permission to punish and control. By focusing on one or other it obscures the role of third parties, including the state or surrounding context, such as social ageism. It is, however, so much part of the common-sense reasoning of the field, that alternative perspectives are almost entirely absent and there is hardly any research on the dynamic of abusive intergenerational relations.

While a division into binary opposites may facilitate action, it has some important disadvantages. First, it tends to divide protagonists into active perpetrators and rescuers and passive victims. It therefore eclipses important debates on the role of resilience in old age (Hildon *et al.*, 2008) and the Foucaultian concept of resistance (Powell and Biggs, 2003). Second, instances of 'wicked people' or 'bad apples' are rare in contexts such as institutional abuse, with mistreatment more likely to be explained as a consequence of dysfunctional organizational cultures (Glendenning, 1993; Goergen, 2007). Were there to be a study of family dynamics and elder mistreatment, its findings would probably be very similar. Third, as noted earlier, mistreatment can often take place between ordinary people who are willing to talk and problem-solve given the right environment, or vulnerable people with mental health and substance abuse problems of their own, placed in challenging situations and succumbing to them (Pillemer and Finkelhor, 1988). A binary opposition reduces the possibilities for empathic understanding and perception of the complexity of relations, themselves key elements in achieving sustainable solutions. Finally, the exclusivity of a binary opposition obscures the influence of social context and structural inequalities that have been elaborated by broader, ecological models (Bronfenbrenner, 1979; Schiamberg and Gans, 2000). Bullying, for example, is difficult to understand without looking to enabling structures, motivating incentives and precipitating processes that contextualize interpersonal conflicts (Salin, 2003). And as Horl (2007) has pointed out, legitimized violence in any setting interacts with questions of official definition and needs to be seen as part of a system of reciprocal relations. A failure to move beyond the binary dyad would be to disrupt understanding of circumstances that permit abuse and facilitate negative stereotyping.

Viewed from this perspective, binary opposites remove ambiguity and resolve discomforting ambivalence so that individuals can remain immersed in systems of unreflective action. A recognition of the two-way nature of intergenerational and age-peer relations, contingent on context, requires a more reflective and nuanced approach. The absence of these themes in the discourse on elder mistreatment is played out in the relative absence of approaches such as family therapy and counselling services (with the notable exception of Norwegian, (Juklestad and Espas, 2006) and Israeli services (Lowenstein and Doron, 2008) or of restorative justice techniques used in other areas (Morrison and Ahmed, 2006)).

Under such circumstances, with a phenomenon that is not containable, yet where one wishes not to slip back to one or other end of a binary contradiction, requires the simultaneous holding in mind of two seemingly incompatible aspects of the same. Recognizing ambivalence offers a mechanism that potentially contains this process. It offers a mature step towards acknowledging a more complex world of multiple perspectives and emotional resilience. To reflectively encounter the dynamic circumstances that lead to and can lead to the avoidance of mistreatment, one must facilitate the possibility of holding both positive and negative emotions about another person in the same clearly defined mental space. This may prevent nominated perpetrators, victims and third parties from engaging in exploitative, abusive or neglectful behaviour as it becomes much less easy to see the age-other instrumentally or neglect to recognize complex interpersonal and moral dilemmas. By contrast, understanding a failure of ambivalence both helps explain how individuals might 'flip' into certain behaviours and raises questions about the circumstances that might trigger and sustain abusive or neglectful relations.

Mistreatment in the absence of Generational Intelligence

Situations that facilitate mistreatment would, by degrees, be situations that induce a state of low GI. First, the state of being abusive may result from an inability to separate out the self and other sufficiently. The other then becomes an extension of the abusing self that can be used instrumentally for one's own ends and to extreme degrees. Second, an encounter with the ageing other is also an encounter with the ageing self, so that by moving away from such an immersive state, protagonists are confronted with what they do not wish to be. They may react by retreating into oppositions outlined previously. The state of being abused may persist out of generational loyalty even though it may produce an inner sense of worthlessness or helplessness, or simply may reflect a physical inability to escape a coercive situation. At a social level, antagonistic expectations arising from wider factors such as conflicting cohort expectations, tensions between care and work roles, changed economic circumstances or policy conditions, may lead to a radical alienation of the other. Part of a solution, would then be to seek out facilitative environments for higher levels of Generational Intelligence: allowing empathic understanding of oneself and other, and when contesting definitions of generation and ageing coexist, enhancing the possibilities for shared problem-solving.

Looking at the genealogy of mistreatment allows us to see how a discipline becomes known to itself. Recognizing ambivalence helps us encounter the other by moving beyond caricature and locating mistreatment in an expanded social environment. Both help us towards generationally intelligent solutions.

To date, the debate has shown characteristics that indicate that it is significantly underdeveloped. Using the vocabulary of Generational Intelligence, it is possible to delineate some of these absences. First, in terms of personal ageing and relations to the self, the field of elder mistreatment is almost entirely immersive. Unlike areas such as child protection and safeguarding (McCluskey and Hooper, 2000), a literature on the effects of working in such potentially disturbing contexts, with older adults, hardly exists. Second, the intergenerational and empathic elements of mistreatment have been superseded by a tendency to unreflectively accept binary descriptions, which polarize the attribution of goodness and badness, and active and passive roles. The problem with this is that, it tends to eclipse the relational character of intergenerational and age-peer activity, rupturing the complexity of relationships over time and context and over-simplifying thought and action. In situations of elder mistreatment, the essentially adult-adult nature of relationships, whether intra-generationally, between partners, or inter-generationally, between adult children and their parents or between older service-users and paid workers, can easily be suppressed, allowing other priorities and preoccupations to dominate the field. A pre-emptive categorization of active and passive or victim and perpetrator roles for example, gives permission to third parties to adopt the role of heroic rescuer, but with little consideration of the sustainability of that approach. In stepping outside this dynamic in order to differentiate the self and see the other more distinctively, high degrees of Generational Intelligence would allow uncomfortable associations and desires, of which we are barely at first aware, to be acknowledged. The fragmentation associated with binary oppositions would put a premium on processes that links the 'them' to the 'us', allow critical perception of structural aspects of generational power, but do not push out diversity and the dynamics of specific circumstances.

Generational Intelligence requires a separation out of self and other within identified boundaries, plus the recognition of the other by holding seemingly incompatible attitudes together in mind at once. This allows negotiated solutions to take shape. This may reduce the likelihood of elder mistreatment, which comes to be seen as a misconceived generational strategy in the absence of perceived alternatives. In order to be understood, mistreatment must also be placed in the context of whether, for example, one trusts the state over and above family members and the implications of disclosure for one's own well-being and those of significant others. Such decisions do not exist in a phenomenological vacuum. They depend upon cohort expectations, historical and life-course experience and a relative willingness to encounter the ambivalence that may arise through them. Without this dimension, mistreatment becomes a particular variety of the unthought-known. It is simultaneously recognized and ignored, becoming a spectacle that offers vicarious revenge on old age plus the comfort of indignation and unreflective action.

9 Workplace and intergenerational relations

Summary

In this chapter, the issue of the workplace and intergenerational relationships is addressed. This issue is related to changes in retirement behaviour and the contention that people would have to work longer to limit the economic impact of changes in population age structure and shrinking workforce.

The chapter presents and analyses the development of the concepts of 'successful ageing', 'productive and active ageing' and the distinction between them, arguing for greater conceptual precision. Relevant gerontological theories related to these concepts – disengagement, activity and continuity theories – are discussed.

What follows is an analysis of one of the main arenas where intergenerational relationships are played out – the workplace. The development of the concept of generations at the workplace is traced, discussing the social dimensions of work, knowledge and ways of working, conflicts and tensions. Finally, looking at Generational Intelligence, as a means of impacting policy and fostering solidarity between generations.

Key points
- the impact of changes in retirement behaviour on generational relations at the workplace;
- the Active, Successful and Productive Ageing perspectives and their implications for work and intergenerational relations;
- related gerontological theories to successful and productive ageing;
- Disengagement, Activity and Continuity theories;
- generations at the workplace – exploring their relationships;
- the social dimension of work for different generational groups;
- knowledge and ways of working – how they evolve for different generations;
- conflicts, tensions and solidarity at the workplace between various generations;
- GI as means of fostering intergenerational solidarity in the arena of the workplace.

Introduction

It has been argued by a wide number of influential international bodies – EU, OECD, UN, World Bank, ILO – that if current trends continue rapid population ageing in industrialized countries is projected to result in labour shortages as well as shortfalls in existing public pensions and health care systems (e.g. Gruber and Wise, 2001; UN, 2002; European Commission, 2005). There is also a growing contention that older persons will need to work longer to limit the economic impact of changes in population age structure. Accordingly, many countries have begun to implement policy changes designed to encourage continued economic activity at older ages (Clark and Quinn, 2002; OECD, 2006).

Recent studies have documented important changes in retirement behaviour, including the slowing or reversal of the trend towards earlier retirement and increases both in gradual retirement and post-retirement returns to the labour force (e.g. Friedberg, 2007; Marshall and Wells, forthcoming).

Despite these trends, the level of labour force participation of older ages is still low. In most industrialized countries – for example, by 2005 in the US it was 20 per cent of the labour force. It was projected that in 2010 in North America, the percentage of 65+ years old still working will be 10 per cent whereas in Europe it will be only 5 per cent (ILO, 2000). This, even though continued work is perceived as significant factor for *productive, active* and *successful* ageing (Dobbs *et al.*, 2007). While some retirement is welcomed and on time, other retirements are involuntary or forced due to the loss of a job, an early retirement incentive, a health problem, mandatory retirement, lack of control with too many job strains or to provide care to a family member (Marshall and Taylor, 2005). Working beyond retirement may give an insight about work behaviour and the relative importance of the workplace for elders and intergenerational relationships. However, many older workers do wish to retire so the wishes of different socio-economic groups and age groups involved should also be considered.

In this chapter we will discuss, analyse and trace the development of the concepts of active, successful and 'productive ageing' and the distinction between them, arguing for greater conceptual precision. Relevant gerontological theories related to these concepts will be outlined. The 2012 European Year of Active Ageing emphasized the importance civil society places on the voices of older people and is also underpinned by the UN Principles for older people to promote independence, care, participation, self-fulfilment and dignity. Then we will focus on 'generations in the workplace', relating to intergenerational dimensions. The aim is to analyse areas of solidarity, conflicts and tensions between generations in work; how to implement effective policies concerning age-related phenomena in the workplace and foster intergenerational relations by utilizing the basic notions of the Generational Intelligence model.

We address generation and the dimensions that constitute the roots of generations in the workplace as a specific combination of cultural-economic – and historical-political (Attias-Donfut, 1988; Mannheim, 1998; Jurkiewicz and Brown, 1998; Gauthier, 2008). These dimensions together shape specific orientations towards the work of each generation.

Active, Successful and Productive Ageing

Attempts to identify the grail of active, successful or productive ageing are well-intended. They recognize the growing numbers of older adults plus medical advances that make many of the decrements previously associated with old age modifiable and in some cases, reversible (Rowe and Kahn, 1987). The debate over successful and productive ageing goes to the heart of ageing studies, and has formed the core of the current disciplinary development of social gerontology. This is because it suggests a means of countering negative stereotyping of older people and increasing their social inclusion, like continued involvement in the workplace.

Posing the question of social ageing in terms of activity, success and/or productivity draws attention to the ways that structural and personal components of identity interact, the techniques used to invent the ageing self and its relationships to other generations. Additionally, the role of public policy in creating an atmosphere that fosters one view of ageing rather than another will be explored.

Ageing policies which emphasized active and successful ageing as a result of being independent and productive were becoming increasingly popular in the late-nineties in North America (Estes and Mahakian, 2001) and parts of Europe (Walker, 2000b; 2006) and were replacing assumptions that old age is a time of dependency and decline. They emphasized the value of work and work-like activities (Biggs, 2001) and of leisure (Katz, 2000). A variety of descriptors have been used almost interchangeably to name this 'new' approach to ageing. For example, a statement submitted to the United Nations World Assembly on Ageing reads:

> A new vision of ageing was proposed that accepts the realities of a fundamental genetically driven bio-molecular process leading to death, but with the prospect of achieving healthy, active, productive, successful and positive ageing to the very end through lifestyle modification and interventions that work.
>
> (Andrews, 1986: 1)

Active and Productive forms have become the most common means of elaborating what 'positive' ageing is all about. Each implies a moral as well as an objective basis on which to grow old, the questions of later life and suggested remedies that can be deployed. While at some levels this may reduce the differential treatment of people based on age, it also constitutes a denial of the special qualities of later life.

In the next section, we will discuss active, successful and productive ageing.

Active and Successful Ageing

The literature on successful ageing, according to Bowling,

> Reveals a wide range of definitions, generally reflecting the academic discipline of the investigator. Biomedical models primarily emphasize physical and

mental functioning as successful aging; socio-psychological models emphasize social functioning, life satisfaction and psychological resources as successful aging. Several studies also identify these factors as the precursors of successful aging. Moreover, research shows that older people consider themselves to have aged successfully, but classifications based on traditional medical models do not.

(2007: 1)

Older people's preferences to remain *active and independent* (Bowling, 2005), together with increasing emphasis on disability-free and healthy-life expectancy in older age, has heightened interest in the promotion of ageing 'successfully' (Gingold, 1999; Fries, 2002). Consequently, definitions of old age are changing, and there is greater recognition that older people are not a homogeneous group (Bowling *et al.*, 2005).

Much of the literature on successful ageing focuses solely on policy initiatives to promote autonomy and independent living in older age. While not underestimating the importance of these to older people, such writings fail to address the question of 'what is successful ageing?' There appears to be little consistency in the definition of the concept, and only two of 16 papers on the topic, published in a supplement of the *Annals of Internal Medicine* in 2003, even attempted to define it (Glass, 2003).

Palmore (1995), in the *Encyclopedia of Aging*, defined successful ageing as survival (longevity), health (lack of disability) and life satisfaction (happiness).

Psycho-social definitions emphasize reaching one's potential, psychological and social well-being (Gibson, 1996), adaptation, control, productivity, social competence and skills, self-mastery, cognitive efficiency and social functioning (e.g. Baltes and Baltes, 1990). Others build on the World Health Organization's definition of health and define it as 'arriving at a level of physical, social, and psychological well-being in old age'(Levkoff *et al.*, 2001).

The Active Ageing – Policy Framework of WHO (2002a) defines active ageing as the process of optimizing opportunities for health, participation and security in order to enhance quality of life as people age. The word 'active' refers to continuing participation in the labour force. The active ageing approach is based on the recognition of the human rights of older people and the United Nations Principles of independence, participation, dignity, care and self-fulfillment. It shifts strategic planning away from a 'needs-based' approach (which assumes that older people are passive targets) to a 'rights-based' approach that recognizes the rights of people to equality of opportunity and treatment in all aspects of life as they grow older.

WHO recommends that active ageing policies should emphasize the importance of participation and the enactment of employment policies and programmes that enable the participation of people in meaningful work as they grow older, according to their individual needs, preferences and capacities (e.g. the elimination of age discrimination in the hiring and retention of older workers). This is in order for people to continue to make a productive contribution to society as they age and maintain independence and autonomy for the longest period of time possible.

Definitions of successful ageing, thus, overlap with concepts of healthy ageing (Vaillant, 2002), positive ageing (Bowling, 1993), productive ageing, active ageing and ageing well, which also lack consistent definitions. There appears to be little interdisciplinary cross-referencing on the topic, increasing conceptual confusion.

MacArthur Foundation studies of successful ageing include social engagement, social roles, participation and activity, social contacts and exchanges and/or positive relationships with others. These variables were reported to be associated with better health, mental and physical functioning (also included in definitions of successful ageing).

Older people also include social roles and activities, social interaction and relationships and social health in their definitions of successful ageing (Bergstrom and Holmes, 2000; Bowling and Dieppe, 2005; Knight and Ricciardelli, 2003; Phelan *et al.*, 2004).

Fisher's (1992; 1995) qualitative samples of older people defined life satisfaction as a precursor of successful ageing. But other older people have defined components of life satisfaction (e.g. happiness) as successful ageing itself (Knight and Ricciardelli, 2003; Palmore, 1979). Regarding the subjective components of life satisfaction, they include zest, resolution, fortitude, relationships between desired and achieved goals, self-concept and mood, including happiness (Neugarten *et al.*, 1961; Valiant, 1990). Life satisfaction has also been the most frequently proposed and investigated component of quality of life (Andrews, 1986; Andrews and Withey, 1976; Campbell *et al.*, 1976) and well-being (Glass, 2003; Walker and Lowenstein, 2009).

In support of a biomedical approach, older people have also emphasized health and functioning in their definitions of successful ageing (Bergstrom and Holmes, 2000; Bowling and Dieppe, 2005; Knight, and Ricciardelli, 2003; Phelan *et al.*, 2004; Tate *et al.*, 2003). Moreover, research shows that, overall, many older people consider themselves to have aged successfully (Bowling and Dieppe, 2005; Strawbridge *et al.*, 2002), but biomedical classifications do not categorize them as such (Strawbridge *et al.*, 2002).

Given this, and the inconsistency with which variables are used as either predictor or constituent variables in the study of successful ageing, advances could be made by grounding the term in older people's multi-dimensional definitions, and building on theoretical approaches. Thus, a definition of successful ageing would include longevity, physical, cognitive, psychological and social health and functioning, effective coping, living circumstances (finances, neighbourhood, etc), interactions with others and overall life satisfaction.

This captures the main approach of each of the models presented, although the models neglected living circumstances. We should consider what are the successful/active amalgams of definitions doing or pointing us towards? Presumably, a reasonably holistic model of what it means to grow old with some degree of satisfaction/social engagement/social usefulness/ should not only be restricted to the workplace and the use of productive ageing but should look at other areas of a person's life. i.e. satisfying family and intimate relations, opportunities for self-fulfillment in the community and in society.

While older people mention effective coping strategies and other psychological factors as part of successful ageing, it is logical that the precursors of these are likely to be possession of various types of resources, like being active in the workplace and other areas, as hypothesized by Baltes and Baltes (1990). Using this approach of being active in different arenas in one's life and trying to maintain autonomy and independence, the different models are complementary to each other, and successful ageing is not only about maintaining good health and functioning, but it is also about coping and remaining in control of one's life in the face of chronic illness (Penrod *et al.*, 2003).

Among the gerontological theories which attempt to outline the variables related to successful ageing we can cite Disengagement, Activity and Continuity theories. Each of which pre-dates the successful ageing debate, but gives important pointers to its constituent and formative parts.

Disengagement, Activity and Continuity theories

The debate between activity and disengagement, as alternative routes through later life, marked the beginnings of modern theorizing in gerontology (Lynott and Lynott, 1996). Activity theory provided the better fit with a moral 'problem-solving' approach adopted by the new discipline. It provided a clear series of objectives that were more easy to measure, making it attractive to the helping professions. Older people needed to maintain their existing activities for as long as possible and replace ones that they had lost with new ones. Whilst much has subsequently been made of the differences between these two explanations of the same Kansas Study (Marshall, 1999), both disengagement and activity theories are a response to the problematization of older people as non-productive: Disengagement theory perceiving the solution for successful ageing to be withdrawal from society, Activity a move to keep doing things for as long as possible. Regardless of its limitations, Activity theory has gained widespread acceptance in professional circles and amongst older people as an antidote to the problem of ageing identity (Gubrium and Wallace, 1990; Biggs *et al.*, 2000). It is, however, unreflective in its attachment to content over explanation (Hendricks and Achenbaum, 1999). What it does do is allow the active body to colonize the sense of self, which is then quantifiable and can be turned into measures and regimes. The world is divided into active elders and those described as 'potentially active'. Activity theory though has been perceived as too narrow in its advocacy of a single lifestyle, given empirical data demonstrating the heterogeneity of older people.

A more popular theory has been Continuity theory (Atchley, 1972), which holds that people who age successfully are those who carry forward their values, lifestyles and relationships from middle to later life. Atchley (1989) shifted the emphasis away from the importance of the volume of activities undertaken for well-being in older age, and stressed adjustment and adaptation to the challenges of ageing by the substitution and redistribution of activities.

In sum, we postulate that a model of successful ageing (see aforementioned) needs to be multi-dimensional, incorporate a lay perspective for social significance, use a continuum rather than dichotomous cut-offs for 'success' and lack of, and distinguish clearly between predictor and constituent variables. It should also be sensitive to differences in opportunities to age successfully and to variations in values between cultures.

Productive ageing

Productive Ageing, which reflects also active aspects, raises the problem of social conformity head-on, by examining the question of ageing through the lens of economic usefulness. Hinterlong *et al.* argue that 'society simply cannot afford to continue to overlook the potential of the older population to serve as a resource for social change and economic growth' (2001: 4). In other words, continue to involve older people in the workplace in order to utilize their social capital.

The policy assumption that older people have become a burden is stood on its head as adherents to Productive Ageing maintain that productivity does not decrease with age. This approach appears radical because it takes as its object the negative stereotyping of older people and is a reaction to intergenerational equity debates in US public policy (Minkler and Robertson, 1991; Collard, 2001). It is pointed out that rather than a steady slide into increasing incapacity, most people are healthier for longer then a decline very quickly before death: labelled a compression of morbidity (Fries, 1990). Also, that there are many advantages for employers hiring older workers, including reliability, prior investment in skills and know-how and company loyalty (Schultz, 1999). There is a basic connection between continued health and productivity in Productive Ageing, because 'engagement in productive behaviour requires a certain level of physical, cognitive and emotional functioning' (Butler *et al.*, 1989).

Productive Ageing originated at the Salzburg conference of 1982 (Butler and Gleason, 1985), at which Betty Friedan, seen by many as the founder of contemporary US feminism, opined 'we can and must express and facilitate our personal and social productivity as we grow older'. Indeed much of the discussion around Productive Ageing has centred on definitions. Caro *et al.* describe Productive Ageing as 'Any activity by an older individual that contributes to producing goods and services or develops the capacity to produce them' (1993: 6) which is similar to Morgan's (1986) definition. Butler and Schechter have proposed in the Encyclopaedia of Aging 'The capacity of an individual or population to serve in the paid workforce, to serve in volunteer activities, to assist in the family, and to maintain himself or herself as independently as possible' (1995: 211). Independence and activity being components of successful ageing.

Thus, Productive Ageing is economic in its foundation and uses efficiency as its core argument. The solution to the problem of ageing is, accordingly, to find a way that older people can be economically useful, either directly, or indirectly. The approach allows the clear measurement of productivity and thus the development of normative judgements, and provides individuals with a clear rational for monitoring their ageing selves. As such, Productive Ageing answers Successful Ageing's liberal avoidance of purpose. The purpose is economic, with the creation of a 'buffer' workforce that can be drawn upon as economic needs demand. Older adults are to find personal value through becoming a pool of surplus labour, although an economic, rather than an ideological justification for the claims of formal productivity have been hard to find (Schultz, 1999). Indeed, the contradiction between exhorting the old and a continued employer preference for younger workers has led to some interesting twists in Rowe and Kahn's (1997) arguments for linking success with productivity. They note, for example the importance of productive engagement to health and continued wellbeing in old age, thus reversing the logic of Butler *et al.*'s (1989) earlier statement, and observe that older people appear not to feel guilty at the rest and leisure that retirement affords. However, as Moody points out, they succinctly link the Productive problematization of old age with the Successful technique of the self: 'the frailty of old age is largely reversible . . . what does it take to turn back the ageing clock? It's surprisingly simple. . . . Success is determined by good old-fashioned hard work' (Rowe and Kahn, 1998: 102; Moody, 2001).

Productive Ageing is a powerful means of reducing ambiguity around the role and place of older people in society. These ideas have become deeply embedded in social policy in both North America (Estes *et al.*, 2001) and in the UK (Biggs, 2001) where work and work-like activities have been presented as turning the burden of an ageing population into an asset and an opportunity. At root, the justification of old age lies in not being a drain on social and economic resources, in which productive ageing is the active justification of 'I can still work' and successful ageing the passive justification of 'look, I'm trying hard not to be a burden on others'.

Biggs (2001) has observed that, whilst positive ageing policies in the UK appear to offer greater choice and flexibility to identity following retirement, they are driven by economic needs based on the changing demography of the British workforce and an unwillingness to meet pension needs. In fact, Productive Ageing provides a powerful counter-blast to the post-modern view of ageing as a time of consumption and associated identity-building. It constitutes not so much an extension of leisure and self-maintenance beyond mid-life as an extension of mid-life values about work to the whole of the adult life-course, which is now seen in terms of workplace values (Sicker, 1994: 165), reflecting also principles from Continuity Theory.

The move towards a 'productive' understanding of Positive Ageing, is not simply a North American phenomenon. It can be seen in European policy towards old age and in national interpretation of the same trends such as in the UK. '*Europe's response to World Ageing: promoting economic and social progress in an ageing world.*' (UN, 2002) recognizes a 'profound transformation in the experience and meaning of old age' based on 'changes in age structure, health and patterns of employment'. And is reflected in, EU, UN and WHO, etc. as noted before. A narrative emerges of flexible retirement, increased longevity with people being healthier for longer and needing to play a valued role in society, if intergenerational solidarity is not to be threatened. Ageing is seen as a site for potential conflict, remedied by work and work-like activities as increased efforts at social inclusion.

However, drawing on the previous discussion of 'success', we can say that the perspectives of productive-active ageing are really too narrow to accommodate the diversity of adult ageing. A core issue here is the degree to which such a dominant view eclipses alternative visions and possibilities in later life. Moreover, because productive and successful ageing are largely concerned with individual conduct, little is said about linking to others and sustaining one's story through others. This has, however been a continuing theme in the literature on the maintenance of self in later life (Ruth and Coleman, 1996). Pillemer *et al.* (2001) have highlighted the value of social integration in the continued well-being and citizenship of older adults. It is, thus, suggested that future policy should seek to enhance integration through connectedness to others and social embeddedness and this would later in this chapter be explored in workplace-intergenerational relations.

We must not ignore 'retirement' as a problematic concept, and think to what stage in the life course is it related? – Should we not rethink the distribution of activity across the life course in addition to being active in the labour market? At the same time, when we focus on the workplace, we should realize that the capacity to work does not necessarily decline before the age of 65 years for most people, as well as motivation to work if it is well-managed (We will examine these issues looking at generations in the workplace.)

Generations in the workplace

Intergenerational relationships are also performed in public arenas such as the workplace, though the rules guiding intergenerational conduct are often implicit.

Using the concept of generation specifically to describe social relations in the workplace is relatively recent. Marshall and Wells (forthcoming) trace the application of the Generations concept to the workplace as far back as a decade ago when a report on *Winning the Generation Game* was published in the UK (UK Civil Service, 2000). The report focused on ways to keep older people in the workforce longer, either as paid workers or volunteers. It used the term generation, without defining it or mentioning generational categories. It only referred to workers 50 years and over, relating to older and younger generations and 'generational attitudes' in terms of the age group (45–64 years). The report used the terms age group and generations synonymously, for example, '. . . engaging them in highly worthwhile activity that helps individuals either of their own age group or across generations' (p. 94). Biggs (2006) criticize this approach, mainly for transposing the aims and ideals of younger onto older generations.

Another report, issued also in 2000 by the Radcliffe Public Policy Center of Harvard University, in partnership with Harris Interactive and Fleetboston Financial, *Life's Work: Generational Attitudes toward Work and Life Integration* was based on data from a cross-sectional survey which discussed the issue in terms of ten-year age categories and confounded the terminology of age group and generation.

A book *Generations at Work* published by Zemke *et al.* (2000), for example, offers a definition of generations which is consistent with Mannheim (1952). However, their operationalization of four defined generations from the Veterans to the Gen Next is inconsistent with most others. Boomers in their book are allocated the cohorts of 1943–60, whereas the common usage is for those born 1946–64. In a series of books, published by Rainmaker Thinking (a consulting firm) they identify Gen Y, Gen X, Cuspers, Boomers and Silents (Martin and Tulgan, 2001; 2002).

When Marshall and Wells continue to explore the issue, they acknowledge that other organizations do not give any definition for the term generation, giving the example of AARP which argues that, in order to combat the coming labour shortage associated with retiring baby boomers, '. . . individuals will need to change their attitudes and traditional assumptions about work and retirement in order to create intergenerational and cohesive work environments' (AARP, 2007: 4). However, except for the baby boomers, the report does not include any other generational categories or labels. Instead, it uses age categories. Another example is the European Commission (2005) report, *Green Paper, Confronting Demographic Change: A New Solidarity between the Generations*, which did not give a definition for the term generation either. Nor did it use generational categories, instead referring to 'young adults', 'older workers', and the 'elderly'. The implications of this imprecision in this context are that it is difficult to distinguish generations in the workplace as it is hard to give specific ages to generations (as was outlined in previous chapters). This means that – it is unclear how 'generation' has been constructed and to what it refers – and therefore when investigating relationships in the workplace we simply have to rely on people's common-sense assumptions.

Till the middle of the last century, the life course as related to work was described as having three major stages: a minimal 'preparation for work' stage, a 'breadwinner' stage and a 'retirement' stage (Cain, 1964: 298). Kohli subsequently described the institutionalization of the life course as 'periods of 'preparation', 'activity' and 'retirement' (1986: 72). In other words, working means being active and productive.

This framework highlights the complexity and variability of the working life course and needed changes (Marshall *et al.*, 2001). Some scholars, though, argue that in recent years the life course has become increasingly individualized and less structured as described earlier. More people follow individualized life-course trajectories with numerous job changes instead of a 'single career', and experience various pre-retirement transitions characterized by bridge jobs, part-time work, etc. (Marshall and Taylor, 2005).

The social dimensions of intergenerational relations in the workplace

Concerning the relations between generations and the factors of cooperation and tensions, scholars often depict the mid-generation as the more protected and the two extreme generations as those who pay the costs of its benefits and security (Giancola, 2006; Martin and Tulgan, 2002). The mid-generation, though, appear a bit envious both of their older colleagues, who still enjoy early-retirement schemes and of the younger ones, more at ease in the digital and flexible society (Edmunds and Turner, 2005; Hughes and O'Rand, 2004). However, the quality of their skills, their position on the labour market, their attitude towards work are important issues. In fact, they are going to be soon the ageing workforce and equitable and sustainable policies for ageing workforce have to be created referring to them. Moreover, for work–life balance, the mid-generation is the most exposed. They are trying to isolate themselves from the younger and the older generation. This might create tensions and conflicts between the different generations as explicated later.

An analysis of the phenomena provided in a European project: 'Social Patterns of Relations to Work'(SPReW; funded under the EU 6th framework programme, 2006) demonstrates that the relations between generations are more complex and that the 'balance of power' is less univocal than it might appear. The project results confirm this complexity and show how different age groups appear to be 'winners' or 'losers' depending on the aspect one considers (e.g. the elders are more exposed to knowledge obsolescence and the younger who just entered the labour market are more exposed to economical stagnation and social insecurity and exclusion) (SPReW project, 2008).

Research of the SPReW project and other scholars distinguishes the *instrumental, social* and *symbolic* dimensions of employment (Paugam, 2000; Nicole-Drancourt and Roulleau Berger, 2001; Riffault and Tchernia, 2002). Briefly, the instrumental dimension refers to 'material' expectations (level of income, security of employment), the social dimension to the importance of human relationships at work and, the symbolic dimension with opportunities for self-development, knowledge acquisition, interest in work content, feeling of success, autonomy and social usefulness. The vision in the pragmatic orientation is that employment is necessary in order to meet personal and family needs. When involvement in work is rather reflexive, work plays a key role in personal identity. Thus, in order to invest in developing stronger solidarity between different generations in the workplace the ability of the individual to 'move' through the various steps to acquire a high Generational Intelligence, as outlined in Chapter 1 of this book, is imperative, taking into account the aforementioned three dimensions. Because one has to move from simple awareness to understanding of other generations and finally being able to behave accordingly.   Data from the SPReW project also shows that other variables such as gender, education, socio-professional groups, economic development and institutional contexts may overwhelm the effect of the 'generation' variable. These data are consistent with major surveys, which analyse attitudes towards work, such as the European Value Survey (EVS), the European Social Survey (ESS) and the International Social Survey Programme (ISSP). Generational differences in this respect are submerged under more dominant definitions of work concern.

Historical and cultural differences among *age groups* do exist, as the surveys show. They result from factors such as the wealth development, which increases post-materialistic orientations; relevance of the work content; polycentric attitude towards life, control of working hours; the increase of tertiary education during the last decades, which is linked to increased expressive orientations; the Information Society, which creates a huge digital divide between last generation and the others; the increasing individualization in identity building; the deregulation of labour markets, which increases job precariousness; the women's employment revolution, which raises the problem of work-life balance and at the same time questions gendered working models.

How far these overall phenomena contribute to 'create' *generations in the workplace?* In a strict sense, according to Mannheim (1952) 'generation units' are a production of historical events: 'individuals who belong to the same generation, who share the same year of birth, are endowed, to that extent, with a common location in the historical dimension of the social process'. They are shaped in opposition to previous generations, they become social movements and agents of change through a process of political self-consciousness. In this sense, not all the age groups are generations and generational boundaries are not the same in all countries.

The SPReW data identified three generations of workers at the workplace: people born before the end of 1950s, people born between this date and the end of 1970s and people born after this last date. In fact, in the second half of the twentieth century, almost everywhere in Europe, an increased protection of labour and the development of welfare systems established a generation of highly protected, strong and collectively represented labour force (the so-called baby-boomers generation). Later on, at the beginning of the 1980s, a new generation of workers emerged, more exposed to unemployment (the so-called X generation). More recently, the necessity for welfare systems to pay pension provisions to a larger population, together with the impact of globalization and the increasing preference for flexible labour markets, produced a generation of more precarious, less collectively represented, less socially protected workers. They are currently defined as the generation Y or the millennial generation (sometimes called the baby-loser generation).

Older workers have a twofold discourse: on the one hand, they describe life in general as being easier for young workers because in the contemporary workplace, relative to their own youth, workers' rights and conditions are more protected, but on the other hand, they describe the employment status of young workers as being extremely difficult compared to what older workers experienced when they entered the labour market. Insecurity, despite the completion of higher education, is seen as the main characteristic of youth trajectories. The life course or trajectory perspective is important in the analysis of intergenerational relationships at work: the differences are rooted in contexts but they also leave their mark. Past history matters in an individual trajectory and past experiences have an impact on future steps, they leave marks that will not disappear spontaneously (Chauvel, 2007b).

We have seen that employment is what gives access to work; it is what defines the conditions in which work will be performed while work refers to the content and organization of activities (Piotet, 2007). This distinction is important because it seems that potential areas of tensions between the generations concern 'employment' rather than 'work'. This section, thus, examined the factors leading to solidarity or tensions in intergenerational relations, in the specific area of employment and work, so we can gain a better understanding of the relationships that diverse generations have, and can analyse the challenges and implications of these changes.

The quality of social relationships is an important aspect of work experience for all age groups, and age does not appear as an obstacle to good working relationships. Generally, age diversity is seen as positive for organizations. In this area, the tension between individualism and solidarity is an important issue, which is most often mentioned by older workers. The workplace is perceived by them as more individualistic than in the past, while solidarity is declining. However, these discourses are very ambiguous because, while saying this, people tell stories that demonstrate the vitality of social bonds in the workplace (Vendramin, 2009).

Discussions about the future of social bonds in the workplace reflect a meeting of two conceptions of the enterprise held by different generations. The majority of older workers' careers were spent in communitarian enterprises, while young workers enter the labour market with images of open organizations, an organizational model, which is promoted in the public sphere. The assumption is that social bonds, solidarity and collective belonging in the workplace are not disappearing but being transformed (Vendramin, 2008).

Knowledge and knowledge transmission

With respect to their portfolios of skills and their working methods, older workers are described as more structured, more logical, more organized, less hyperactive, more serene. They bring their wisdom to bear in their daily work. These attributes are seen as the product of experience. By contrast, young workers are described (by themselves as well) as excited, chatty, impulsive. Older workers are not considered as less efficient than their younger counterparts. Efficiency is seen as the product of time and experience.

Knowledge capital and knowledge transfer are key issues, with the different generations having different viewpoints. Some young workers say they must take the initiative and ask questions to older workers; the exchange of knowledge is not spontaneous, though. For others, knowledge-sharing is natural and comes automatically through cooperation, when the organization and work rhythms allow such cooperation, and when young workers are not confined to peripheral tasks. Knowledge transmission is not only a matter of age, all newcomers are in learning situations. If experience belongs to older workers, young workers seem to be more at the cutting edge of new working methods. Finally, transmission of knowledge is not seen as a unidirectional phenomenon, it also flows from younger to older workers.

Managing age diversity at work, rather than reinforcing age segregation through targeted policies and measures that reinforce stereotypes, can support knowledge transmission in both directions, mutual recognition and trust and foster social cohesion (Cheren, 2000; Dobbs, 2007; Hanks and Icenogle, 2001). Such avenues are important for encouraging solidarity and activating the pathway towards a successful and sustainable high GI. However, we should consider the possibility that more awareness of generations may initiate social tensions. (Cook Ross, 2004)

Solidarity, conflicts and tensions

Research highlights the role of institutional factors (education system, the family, the labour market regulation, the welfare state model) in drawing boundaries among age groups. Thus, young workers (< 30 years) are more exposed to precariousness and unemployment but they benefit from a positive educational and digital differential. The adult generation (30 to 50 years) usually enjoys a stable position in the labour market but is more exposed to the difficulties related with keeping together career expectations and family care. The elder generation (> 50 years) – when they are still at work – enjoys the best wages and security and the highest representation by trade unions, but they are the most exposed in case of company restructuring because of deskilling (e.g. Cheren, 2000; Marshall and Wells, forthcoming).

Between the two extreme groups a certain amount of tension, more than conflict, was evident which may be related to: a kind of incommunicability in approach to work, due to a diversity in the mix of competencies and especially in 'languages' (digital vs analogical, global vs local); the changing meaning attributed to work in different economic and social periods, where different work values are prevailing: young people often don't agree with old workers' centrality of work, while the old workers complain about apparent young people disaffection to work; the psychological distance between ages: young workers appear both more cynical and more passionate towards work, while old workers often solved the cognitive dissonance between attainment and expectations telling their work story as a success history. This evidence suggests that misunderstandings are both a matter of age and of generations (Vendramin, 2009; Marshall, and Wells, forthcoming)

The different generations have to share labour market opportunities with former generations, so there will necessarily be losers and winners. There is a specific balance of weakness and strength for all generations. In such a context, intergenerational relations are becoming a key issue for social cohesion and intergenerational solidarity, for integration of all generations in the workplace but also, for employers and employees, to take benefits from age diversity and try to minimize tensions and conflicts.

Data show that a real strong conflict among generations is not observed (e.g. Giancola, 2006), though possible tensions can be foreseen, especially for two reasons: the objective working conditions of the last generation, in terms of employment opportunities, social security and collective representation have greatly changed; particularly in manufacturing, the traditional cooperation at the workplace based on everyday practice and knowledge transmission between old and young workers does not work anymore, due to the sharp divide occurring between old industrial skills and new digital skills (e. g. Marshall and Taylor, 2005). Moreover, the research highlights that objective critical aspects exist for each generation (or age group). In particular, the mid-generation faces specific 'generational' problems (as for their harder involvement in family commitments), while the old 'lucky' ones are the most exposed to company reorganization. As a consequence, every group has different expectations as far as the quality of working life (Vendramin, 2009).

Some scholars further argue that generational conflicts in the workplace:

> may be more myth than reality, as a growing body of independent research and expert opinion shows that concerns about a generation gap have been overstated and, surprisingly, the theory behind it has some gaps in logic that raise serious questions about its value.
>
> (Giancola, 2006: 32)

This is related to the idea that work's domination of life gives way to a multi-dimensional approach to life in which other areas: place, family status, social status, and so forth are also important. Thus, peoples' identities encompass many selves, as Vincent argues:

> As with other statuses, generations are fluid{mdash}boundaries solidify and relax, are appropriate in different contexts and not in others, and are nested into broader and narrower categories. These contexts are not simply the broad historical times of change identified by Mannheim and Turner but local and specific and emergent from personal biography and family and community situation. . . . Generational identities are contingent on specific social situations in which they become meaningful and not tied to a biological rhythm.
>
> (Vincent, 2005: 584)

To sum up, even though a certain amount of tension more than conflict was found to exist between different generational groups in the workplace but much of the assumed conflict was found to be a myth. However, we should also consider specific work roles, specific working contexts and specific social situations where various generations meet,

Fostering intergenerational relations – Generational intelligence

One should not only focus on the negative outcomes of generational differences in the workplace, but also on sources of strength. For example, intergenerational transfers of knowledge are important in maintaining the institutional knowledge of an organization. There is the transmission of new technical knowledge from younger to older generations and intergenerational mentoring can flow in both directions and provide positive outcomes for intergenerational solidarity. We would argue that sustainable intergenerational relationships will need to rely on increased levels of generational insight, empathy and mutually negotiated action. Thus, when different generations become aware of the skills and knowledge of other generations and start to understand their needs they might be able to put themselves in the position of the age-other. Organizations that lack generational or age group balance can face serious problems in areas such as succession planning and the provision of career opportunities (Howe and Strauss, 2007).

A recent study on generations in the IT workplace showed that the information technology workers invoke a generational discourse in relation to personal identity formation and in shared discourse at the firm level. The 'generational affinities' that form the basis of this discourse are related to the fact that people of different birth cohorts were immersed to varying degrees and in different ways in the succession of computer technologies that emerged over the past decades (McMullin *et al.*, 2007). As Marshall and Wells (forthcoming) discuss, this approach could be usefully applied in other work domains. For example, in transportation, we might expect to find generational differences following introduction or dissemination of new transportation modalities such as the use of jet aircraft or online reservation and ticketing systems. However, there should be a trade-off between the generations and intergenerational collaboration needs to be a two-way street, where each generation can learn and benefit from the others knowledge and expertise which will foster intergenerational solidarity.

Most people in work after 50 years would consider working longer, but more flexibly. What older people want from work are: respect and identity; ability to use skills and knowledge; purpose and meaning; social engagement; money; reduced stress – health and work-life balance; and control and flexibility. And for younger workers they need support, they need to 'learn the ropes' and acquire organizational understanding, and learn process and seeing the 'big picture'. In other words, the exchange has to be reciprocal or it won't work.

Thus, the challenges are: to redistribute work; redefine work; improve the quality of work; recognize heterogeneity of individuals and generations; and promote lifelong learning. On the economic level – trying to solve the problems of a shrinking workforce, especially in many European countries, and trying to accommodate generations 'sandwiched' between the demands of younger and older dependents? We should help working families – what the Australians call 'the battlers' – with young kids, dual careers, uncertainty and can't afford the housing ladder who fulfil multiple roles that impact their work lives. In order to achieve this, different generations have to acquire a high Generational Intelligence in order not only to understand another generational needs but also be able to 'give up' some of their needs to better accommodate the needs of another generation.

In order to enhance generational solidarity at the workplace and based on empirical research, institutional and company measures should be oriented at: re-balancing the *specific weakness* of each generation on the labour market (i.e. more social protection for young workers, more retraining for the elders), thus avoiding the risk of a future increased intergenerational unbalance; answering the *expectations* of each group i.e. change in work organization for young people, more family-friendly policies at the company level for mid-generations, humanization of work for old workers; improving *understanding* between different age-groups by encouraging mutual mentoring and fostering intergenerational cooperation at work, through the articulation of career paths and the modularization of training systems (Kupperschmidt, 2000).

To conclude, we have to realize that in order to use the model of Generational Intelligence in the workplace arena, we need to find ways of 'getting the balance right' between the different generational groups, and imprint the value and usefulness of reciprocal understanding and skill-sharing. Furthermore, we should resist narratives that create an unbalanced work-life relationship or skew the answer to work (as age-skewed) as the main form of social inclusion. Dominant ideologies in society privilege work above other forms of intergenerational activity. However, intergenerational relations provide the context within which individuals grow and mature and is reflected in such relations taking place at work. Relations at work, though, are more complex than is often the case as portrayed in current policy/theory. Relations at work need to seek complementarity and Generational Intelligence is a key process in achieving some form of intergenerational reciprocity and solidarity at work. It is not simply enough to become self-consciously aware of one's own and another's life-course priorities as related to work and other areas. It is also important to achieve a rapport between them, and find ways of negotiating a complementary relationship that can be sustained over time. It has, in other words, to work for both parties and to be able to last.

As outlined in Chapter 1, Generational Intelligence not only focuses on a single person's or generations' perspective but also creates the possibility of a space emerging, in which multiple generational viewpoints can be taken into account. A space for younger and older workers to exchange ideas and knowledge and learn from one another, this gives the opportunity for a process of pragmatic negotiation to take place and to be sustained over time.

10 Intergenerational relations in the community

Summary

The Madrid International Plan of Action on Ageing (2002), dealt with the topic of how to create more favourable environments for ageing and foster intergenerational solidarity in various spheres, including in communities, if our 'societies are to be for all ages' (Sidorenko and Walker, 2004). One possible avenue in which solidarity between generations can grow is by developing intergenerational community programmes.

Accordingly, this chapter will analyse the concept of 'A society for all ages', discussing the components of such perspective which include facets of ageing converging on this idea: 1) The situation of older persons; 2) Lifelong individual development; 3) Multigenerational relationships; and 4) Development and ageing populations. It will be followed by a discussion and analysis of intergenerational community programmes, the rationale for their creation; looking at different types of programmes: those where younger are serving old, old are serving young, old and young are serving together and intergenerational shared sites. The benefits to different participants in such programmes will be analysed, leading to the activation of Generational Intelligence within such programmes and future challenges.

Key points

- the meaning of 'A society for all ages' as declared by the United Nations;
- the development of intergenerational community programmes and their goals;
- discussing different types of programmes, goals and participants;
- benefits to participants of different generational groups;
- activating GI within such programmes in the framework of community programmes.

Introduction

In June 2000, the United Nations General Assembly decided to convene the Second World Assembly on Ageing, in order to present recommendations concerning how to best combine socio-economic development and demographic ageing. The approval of the Madrid International Plan of Action on Ageing in 2002, dealt also, with the topic of how to create more favourable environments for ageing; how to foster intergenerational solidarity in various spheres, including in communities, in order to implement the recommendation for 'societies are to be for all ages', as proposed by the United Nations since 1995.

One possible avenue in which solidarity between generations can grow is by developing intergenerational programmes. As Villar states:

> The term *inter-generational* implies the involvement of members of two or more generations in activities that potentially can make them aware of different (generational) perspectives. It implies increasing interaction, cooperation to achieve common goals, a mutual influence, and the possibility of change (hopefully, a change that entails improvement).
>
> (2007: 115–16; italics added for emphasis)

Bengtson's domains of familial intergenerational solidarity (Bengtson *et al.*, 1990), which were discussed in detail in Chapter 6, also serve as powerful indicators of solidarity between generations in the larger community. Advocates of a society for all ages uphold ideals of positive intergenerational sentiment (affectual solidarity), shared values (consensual solidarity), and an opportunity structure that favours intergenerational contact (structural solidarity) and reflects a commitment to civic roles and obligations (normative solidarity). Such programmes can, thus, help reduce discrimination against older persons, be a source of intergenerational solidarity and can be suitable instruments for increasing the integration and cohesion in societies.

A central issue is how to foster social change which will enable the creation of 'a *society for all ages*', as the Madrid plan calls for. One route is to increase and organize the opportunities available to people from one generation to relate to people from other generations, and enable different generations to make use of such opportunities and thus, to increase intergenerational interaction and the discovery of common goals. The more interactions between various generational groups and more exposure to personal knowledge and capabilities, more positive relations between generations could be developed. Then some of the barriers currently preventing our societies from truly being societies for all ages will be demolished.

Attitudes indicating presence or absence of intergenerational community solidarity should be reflected in a generations' support for programmes and policies that directly benefit another age group. For example, data show quite a high public support for welfare programmes primarily serving older adults (such as Social Security or other pension programmes) (Cook and Barrett, 1992), which may reflect indicators of consensual solidarity. Silverstein and Parrott (1997) also reported support across cohorts of Social Security, but younger persons were less likely to view cutting elder programmes as a violation of the public good.

Accordingly, this chapter will review the basic idea of 'a *society for all ages*', focusing on intergenerational programmes in various communities, presenting examples of best practices and what are the lessons we can learn. The main components of such programmes will be identified, including their benefits for the different generations participating and their role in social policies required creating a *society for all ages*. Finally, looking at how the Generational Intelligence perspective can be activated within such programmes to increase intergenerational solidarity among different generations in society.

A society for all ages

The roots of this concept are found in the World Summit for Social Development, held in Copenhagen in 1995. According to Chapter IV of the Summit report, on Social Integration: 'The aim of social integration is to create a society for all, in which every individual, each with rights and responsibilities, has an active role to play' (United Nations, 1995: 66).

The conceptual framework defined four facets of ageing converging on the idea of a *society for all ages*: 1) The situation of older persons; 2) Lifelong individual development; 3) Multigenerational relationships; and 4) Development and ageing populations (Sanchez *et al.*, 2007). These four facets will be briefly elaborated.

The situation of older persons

The Vienna Plan (1982) made older persons the object of different ageing policies and the first World Assembly (1983) convened to establish an international plan of action aimed at guaranteeing the economic and social security of older persons, as well as opportunities for them to contribute to the development of their nations (United Nations, 1983). The idea was to create a 'new ageing culture'.

Lifelong individual development

This new approach to ageing, which rejects the idea of *old age* as a specific stage of life, opened the door for support for healthy ageing, closely followed by active ageing, which had been discussed in our previous chapter. Societies must be *for all ages* because all their members, regardless of age, must be able to continue contributing to their well-being, providing that societies, in turn (including families and communities), provide persons of all ages with all the necessary support so that their participation becomes actually feasible, fostering foresight and self-confidence.

Multigenerational relations

A long-living society is also a society in which different generations have to live together and strive towards common goals. This opens the door to possible new forms of interaction between generations in families, communities and society.

The '*society for all ages*' concept is multigenerational by definition. Moreover, it must be intergenerational. Collaboration between generations is a key factor in the maintenance of social structures capable of responding to the needs of older persons; needs which, are linked to the needs of people of other ages. It fosters independence and interdependence.

Development and ageing populations

According to Sidorenko (2007: 6) 'the idea was to harmonize an ageing population with continued socioeconomic development'. The key to this fourth dimension was the *(inter)dependence of the population*. What does this mean? That ageing can only become a developmental factor if we collaborate with one another, maintaining a kind of contract according to which it is acceptable for all of us. This is where the macro and micro adjustments in a changing world are made.

Finally, two aspects which have also been referred to in other dimensions of the concept are: the need to favour multigenerational sharing and promote active ageing at the site of residence.

In the conclusions of the Second World Assembly on Ageing (Madrid, 2002), the United Nations recognized 'the need to strengthen solidarity between generations and intergenerational partnerships, keeping in mind the particular needs of both older and younger ones, and encourage mutually responsive relationships between generations' (United Nations, 2002: 4). One way of achieving this is to 'encourage and support traditional and non-traditional multigenerational mutual assistance activities in families, the neighborhood and the community'(United Nations, 2002: 18). In this respect, intergenerational programmes are appropriate instruments for encouraging and strengthening solidarity between generations.

Intergenerational community programmes

Intergenerational community programmes started about in the 1970s in the US in order to correct what was then perceived as a threat for its society: the growing distance and confrontation between different generations as a result of changes in the labour market which created and/or strengthened stereotypes about the older population. The second phase, up to the 1990s, and also in North America, was characterized by activating intergenerational programmes to approach social problems related to cultural, social and economic needs, targeted towards mitigating the problems affecting two highly vulnerable populations, children/ youngsters and older persons. Finally, the third phase, involves the growing use of such programmes for community development in an attempt to revitalize communities which, in the long run, could be expected to re-connect different generations. This objective is the most consistent with the construction of a *society for all ages*.

At the end of this decade, such programmes started to grow with some force in Europe. They appeared in response to problems such as the difficult integration of immigrants. For example in the Netherlands social cohesion is one of the key concepts of local social policy, where special attention is paid to those groups who maintain little to no social contact or amongst whom tensions arise: different age groups and communities with different ethnic and cultural backgrounds. Thus, a neighbourhood-reminiscence programme was developed, using memories and stories of neighbourhood residents in order to promote exchanges, mutual understanding and respect between different age- and cultural-groups (Mercken, 2003). The programme had been developed in response to political issues related to inclusion and the new roles to be played by the elderly in the United Kingdom (UN, 2002; Hatton-Yeo, 2006), or the perception of a crisis affecting traditional family solidarity and family obligations towards elders and interest in fostering active ageing, like in Spain where elders and youth are integrated in one community setting (Sanchez, 2007).

Late in the last century, efforts emerged designed to move the focus of intergenerational practice from serving individuals to a potentially wider impact taking a neighbourhood or community-based approach. These initiatives ranged from a country-wide effort like that described previously in the Netherlands (Mercken, 2003) to community-based developments in the United States. These efforts are combining best practices from the fields of community development, environmental protection and human development. Going beyond a single programme, these approaches were intended to engage people where they live their lives and prevent old and young from being marginalized (Sanchez *et al.*, 2007).

Sanchez and his colleagues present some of the definitions used in the literature for intergenerational programmes: 'Activities or programs that increase cooperation, interaction and exchange between the members of any two generations. They involve sharing skills, knowledge and experience between young and older people' (Ventura-Merkel and Liddoff, 1983).

Intergenerational programmes

> Bring together both the young and old to share experiences that benefit both populations. Intergenerational programs are designed to engage non-biologically linked older and younger persons in interactions that encourage cross-generational bonding, promote cultural exchange, and provide positive support systems that help to maintain the wellbeing and security of the younger and older generations.
>
> (Newman, 1997: 125)

> Intergenerational programmes are vehicles for the purposeful and ongoing exchange of resources and learning among older and younger generations for individual and social benefits.
>
> (Hatton-Yeo and Ohsako, 2001)

> Activities or programmes that increase cooperation, interaction and exchange between people from any two generations. They share their knowledge and resources and provide mutual support in relations benefiting not only

individuals but their community. These programmes provide opportunities for people, families and communities to enjoy and benefit from a *society for all ages.*

(Generations United, undated)

Three aspects, however, are found as the common denominators in all these definitions: a) People from different generations participate b) Participation in an intergenerational programme involves activities aimed at goals which are beneficial for all those involved (and hence to the community in which they live) and c) In all these programmes participants maintain relations based on sharing.

Rather than artificially segregating people by age cohort which reflects institutionalizing generational separation (Kohli, 1996), intergenerational programmes offer an alternative view of a world that honours all ages, all generations and their abilities. Such programmes, however, 'focus on non-kin relationships and family relationships that skip a generation' (Hanks and Pomzetti, 2007: 8–9). Additionally, 'Intergenerational programs owe their existence to the convergence of a number of social, economic, and political factors, as well as to a unique synergy that seems to exist between older adults and young people' (Newman *et al.*, 1997: 3). Intergenerational contact, though, does not always have positive effects (Aday *et al.*, 1993) so we must attend to not only the structure and availability of intergenerational contact but also the quality of the contact setting (Schwartz and Simmons, 2001).

As people age, many long to be engaged – they want to give back to their communities. In a 2001 Civic Ventures survey of 600 older Americans aged 50 years to 75 years, including 300 volunteers and 300 non-volunteers, 56 per cent of baby boomers said civic engagement will be at least fairly important in their retirement. Working with children was found to be the most appealing volunteer activity among older adults, with 35 per cent seeing that as most enjoyable, followed by service to religious organizations, other seniors and hospitals. Intergenerational programmes provide a tremendous opportunity for such activities. In California, for example, older volunteers are involved with socially isolated young people living in low-income neighbourhoods in after-school programmes (Adler, 2003).

Throughout life, mental and physical health is affected by the presence, absence and quality of ties to other people. Intergenerational programmes are about building meaningful ties that connect people. Intentional, well-thought out Intergenerational programmes allow people of all ages and abilities to share their talents and resources, supporting each other in relationships that benefit both them and society.

Intergenerational practice

Intergenerational practice has developed over the years into a more systematic effort to address social problems. For example: providing extra support for low-income children; teaching a person of another age a new skill; working together to protect the environment (e.g. Adler, 2003; Newman *et al.*, 1999; Ohsako, 2002).

Originally designed simply to bring young and old together, intergenerational initiatives now encourage each generation to contribute. Intergenerational programmes involving cooperation, as opposed to competition, as youth and elders work towards a common goal which is central to positive contact. In fact, cutting-edge work melds the principles of intergenerational practice with community development, involving many generations to improve civic life (Osborne and Bullock, 2000). Not only do intergenerational programmes encourage community participation, but they also promote healthy ageing among all generations. Studies have shown that older adults who volunteer regularly with children burn 20 per cent more calories per week, experience fewer falls and rely less on canes (e.g. Maccallum *et al.*, 2006).

Elders, especially the young-old (65–80 years) can remain productive and valued as contributing members of society. They can also learn from young people and forge new friendships. Intergenerational opportunities can give older adults a chance to pass along the value of volunteerism and community involvement to younger ages. They also provide a way to convey culture and traditions to new generations. As one retired shipyard worker said after completing an oral history project, 'I never knew my life had meaning until now.'

Young people engaged in intergenerational programmes gain an awareness and appreciation of ageing, often reporting they do not fear ageing as much as those who have not shared time with elders like in after-school programmes.

If contact between generations becomes an optimal way to support intergenerational solidarity, contact needs to be voluntary (Jarrott and Bruno, 2007). Some children and seniors will need time to acclimatize to the intergenerational setting if they have had limited contact with the other generation.

Gaining awareness of another generation is the first step in the process of acquiring Generational Intelligence like when youngsters meet older volunteers in an after-school programme or in a shared site of a day care for elders operating within a school. In addition, they benefit from interpersonal relationships with people of different age groups, who can provide guidance, wisdom, support and friendship and can thus advance to the second step of Generational Intelligence by differentiating self from other but at the same time understanding the needs and abilities of other generations.

Types of intergenerational programmes

Developing intergenerational programmes, one must think 'outside the box' and adopt an intergenerational lens. What is the potential to engage people across the ages? How many people would think, for example, that an 82-year-old could lead a teenage exercise class? That's what happens at an upstate New York activity centre. Who would think that a 12-year-old would want to help deliver meals on wheels and perform home safety inspections for shut-in elders? Yet older adults in Florida benefit each day from the efforts of children and youth references for these points.

Intergenerational programmes range from programmes based on the idea of *doing something for others*, whether they be children, youngsters or older persons,

to programmes consisting of *learning with* in which collaboration and mutual benefit are paramount (Manheimer, 1997). While there are many variations on the
theme, most intergenerational programmes fit into one of the four types outlined
later, each providing various benefits to its participants.

Young serving old

Young people who volunteer do better in school than peers who do not. They have
a sense of purpose and are more likely to feel like they belong. Youth involved
in intergenerational programmes may be teaching older adults to use computers,
mentoring older immigrants as they prepare for citizenship tests, assisting home-
bound elders with home projects or delivering meals on wheels.

As summarized by Marx *et al.* (2004), the benefits for children participating
in intergenerational programmes include positive changes in perceptions of and
attitudes to older persons, and increased empathy towards them, as well as more
knowledge about ageing. Additionally, such involvement enhanced pro-social
conduct as sharing, increased self-esteem, greater school attendance, better attitudes to school, better behaviour at school and better bargaining skills and social
relations.

Old serving young

Older adults of all abilities can support children and youth, as well as their families. Intergenerational programmes provide a reason to get out of bed in the morn-
ing – whether it is to tutor a child, offer support over the telephone after school,
lead a nature walk or support a family with a special needs child. For example,
according to their involvement in a volunteer programme in a school, mentors
claimed to have increased their self-esteem, be in better health and enjoy the satisfaction of feeling productive (Newman and Larimer, 1995). In another evaluation study by Fried *et al.* (2002), it was found that after four months of intensive
participation, in a programme in schools which relate the local retired community
to primary school children – the older persons showed a reduction in depressive
symptoms, watched less television every day, developed more problem-solving
skills and increased their mobility.

Young and old serving together

Intergenerational programmes in which young people and older adults work
together to meet real needs can bring tremendous benefits to the community
(Generations United, 2002). At the same time, young and old gain an appreciation
for one another when working together to plan events, research and debate ballot
measures, monitor the environment or perform in an orchestra or theatre troupe,
for example. Intergenerational practice helps to increase tolerance, the level of
comfort and closeness between young and old, helping to demolish clichés and
myths related to the ageing process (Manheimer, 1997).

Intergenerational shared sites

As communities confront the need to provide services across the lifespan, more innovative cities and towns are using their limited resources to connect generations rather than separate them. Intergenerational shared sites are programmes where children, youth and older adults receive services at the same site (Generations United, 2006). While these intergenerational shared sites may vary in structure, their common thread is that they provide at least two programme components: one that serves children or youth and one that serves older adults. These individuals interact regularly during the day in scheduled intergenerational activities, as well as informally when their paths cross. Intergenerational shared sites vary in structure and include models such as a seniors' centre in a public school, an adult and child day care, or an after-school programme in a continuing care retirement community. Shared site intergenerational programmes are uniquely positioned to connect the generations because they provide ongoing services concurrently to children and seniors. Care programmes are the most common shared site setting.

In recent years, there are a number of intergenerational programmes which are described in detail by Jarrot and Bruno (2007). Programmes successful for bringing intergenerational activities to schools and communities were highlighted in a special issue of *Generations*, guest edited by Nancy Henkin and Eric Kengson (1998–1999). These programmes included interventions in after-school care (Larkin, 1998–1999), immigration (Skilton-Sylvester and Garcia, 1998–1999) and families at risk (Power and Maluccio, 1998–1999).

The type of activity performed in an intergenerational programme varies depending on where the interactions take place, the participants involved, the time they spend together, etc. There are, however, some points in common which can be underlined (Kuehne, 2003): activities are usually related to the individual needs of each group of participants and the programmes aim to benefit the generations involved.

Quality intergenerational programmes reflect a balanced relationship and understand that the key element is reciprocity between generations. Each age group gives, and receives, through the interaction. Reciprocity was also found to be an important element in intergenerational family relationships, benefiting different generations (Lowenstein *et al.*, 2007) as well as in intergenerational programmes where young and old work together, as outlined earlier (Manheimer, 1997). Provision of varied intergenerational programmes opportunities supports high levels of voluntary intergenerational contact and increases the range of needs that can be addressed intergenerationally. Programmes that bring the generations together also promote active ageing – a concept summed up by the International Council on Active Ageing as 'engaged in life' and which was discussed in detail in the previous chapter.

Because professionals working with youth and older adults typically have expertise limited to one generation or the other, cross-training is recommended for intergenerational practitioners (Jarrott *et al.*, 2006). Such training typically addresses developmental characteristics of the two (or more) age groups, the purpose and anticipated benefits and challenges of intergenerational programmes, and evidence-based practices for connecting the generations.

Evaluation studies identify four factors related to intergenerational program activities that seem to be critical to their success:

1) Activities should be related to the individual needs of those in one or, preferably, both participant groups (i.e., young and old).
2) Activities can be created for purposes that are both related to the individuals involved and for the benefit of others as well (e.g., community).
3) Intergenerational program participants should have a role in planning activities; and
4) A clear link should exist between program goals, activities and research and/ or evaluation outcome measures.

(Kuehne, 2003)

Outcomes of intergenerational programmes

Evidence has supported the conclusion that positive interactions between age groups can influence attitudes about ageing and older adults positively (Mosher-Ashley and Ball, 1999) – for example, Chamberlain *et al.* described the value of intergenerational programmes for helping to change age-related stereotypes. They note:

> It is generally only in the context of educational programmes about ageing or gerontology and intergenerational programmes where children can perceive an idea of ageing as the development of an active life of service, seeing older persons as community resources even at an advanced age.
>
> (1994: 196)

Yet, there is another perspective, one that emphasizes a view of older adults as societal assets. Freedman (1999), for example, describes the population ageing trend as an 'opportunity to be seized.' Moreover, the participants in intergenerational programmes develop skills which generate expected changes – changes in themselves, changes in their organizations and changes in the communities in which they live. In programmes aimed at developing a *community for everyone*, the participants learn important leadership skills including, for instance, how to effectively form strategic alliances with key organizations and individuals.

Having older adults present and playing constructive roles in the lives of children and youth, for example, can be of pivotal importance in providing needed social and emotional support and promoting healthy development (Taylor *et al.*, 1999). Older adults find, for example, that volunteering provides a venue for better health and well-being. Research has shown that volunteers have greater longevity, higher functional ability, lower rates of depression, less use of canes and less incidence of heart disease (Civic Ventures, 2005).

There are efforts to programmatically bring children and youth together with older adults. Such programmes are found in settings including schools, community organizations, hospitals and places of worship. They mobilize the talents, skills, energy and resources of older adults (as well as young people) in service to people of other generations (Henkin and Kingson, 1998/99). Moreover, they have been found to be a practical, effective means for diminishing ageist stereotypes, improving services for children, youth and older adults, and strengthening community support systems. Within such programmes, the process of Generational Intelligence can be activated by continued interactions between the different generations, continued contributions and collaboration. Such a process enables raising awareness of other generations, understanding 'the other' and being able to sometimes give up their needs in order to answer the needs of another generation.

Intergenerational programmes have demonstrated capacity to support children's (e.g. Marx *et al.*, 2004) and elders' well-being (Hayes, 2003; Jarrott and Bruno, 2003; 2007), reduction in depressive symptoms for elders (Fried *et al.*, 2000); improve community and attitudes towards intergenerational contact among staff (Jarrott *et al.*, 2004), contribute to caregiver benefits (Gigliotti *et al.*, 2005) and provide cost-effective care (Chamberlain *et al.*, 1994). Older adults have been used as mentors to youth at risk of drug use and dropping out of school (Taylor *et al.*, 1999) and as living historians addressing students' curriculum (e.g. Bales *et al.*, 2000; Meshel and McGlynn, 2004).

Outcomes for individuals of intergenerational programmes include: improved attitudes towards other generations, increased involvement in community improvement efforts, increased interaction across ages and culture, and increased service utilization. Specific benefits for older persons range from individual ability to cope with mental disease and increased motivation, to relational aspects – making friends with young people, and benefits for the community – reintegration in community life (Maccallum *et al.*, 2006). Benefits for children and young people of intergenerational learning-service, for example, provides participants with opportunities to develop qualities such as initiative, flexibility, openness, empathy and creativity and to obtain a sense of social responsibility as well as to the potential benefit of intergenerational programmes for enhancing resiliency in youth (Goff, 2004).

Outcomes for organizations include: increased collaboration around issues, increased awareness and utilization of intergenerational approaches, and increased interaction between service providers and clients. Outcomes for communities include: increased resident awareness and appreciation of local history and environmental (natural and built) resources, increased local participation in community development decision-making processes, and the degree to which real community needs are met, such as increased safety, improved transportation and the protection of natural resources such as lakes. It also increases the level of civic vitality in the communities in which programmes are established (e.g. Kaplan and Chadha, 2004), Intergenerational programmes form part of a larger intergenerational strategy to build more inclusive and involved communities providing more care, in which all the generations can give and receive support. This can be found in an effort to renew the 'social contract'(Henkin and Kingson, 1999).

Intergenerational programmes have been found to affect older adults' views of young people. Older adults are most likely to adopt positive views about young people when they have a chance to see youth behaving in competent ways, when contact is prolonged, and when they have opportunities for discussion and reflection with the youth participants (Zeldin *et al.*, 2000).

For older adults such programmes create 'productive ageing' opportunities, defined as activities which promote a sense of purpose, involvement in paid and volunteer activities, and that contribute to independent living outcomes. There seems little question that intergenerational programme environments can be ones in which children construct knowledge about a great many things, including the diverse and rich experiences and knowledge of older adult participants.

In general, the various intergenerational programmes described earlier improve intergenerational communication within families, leading to enhanced understanding about the experiences, relationships, roles and responsibilities of people in other generations. However, how to sustain such programmes? Indicators of intergenerational community programme sustainability include: (a) leadership competence, (b) effective collaboration, (c) understanding the community, (d) demonstrating programme results, (e) strategic funding, (f) staff involvement, and (g) programme responsivity. Beyond these markers, intergenerational advocates share the responsibility to disseminate their experiences in order to shape future practice and policy. Intergenerational strategies evolve to address the ever-changing circumstances of societies (Jarrot, 2007).

Individual development and fostering Generational Intelligence

Many practitioners working with older adults in senior centres, retirement residences, nursing homes and other settings see intergenerational programmes as an opportunity for older adults to develop themselves, and to share their accumulated knowledge and care with a younger and often eager audience. For example, psychologists such as Erik Erikson (1959) have written about the important role that the concept of 'generativity' plays in adult development. Generativity involves guiding and caring for those in the next generation, and while generativity can appear in many different forms (McAdams and De St. Aubin, 1998), intergenerational programmes have long been viewed from the conceptual perspective of older adults fulfilling their own developmental needs, while simultaneously contributing to their environments and others' development as well (e.g. Kuehne, 1992; Van Der Ven, 1999).

Activity theory has also been applied to older adults' involvement in intergenerational programmes. This theory was developed in North America and basically suggests that as ageing adults lose various social roles in society, they maximize their sense of well-being, life satisfaction and self-concept when the lost roles are replaced with new ones (e.g. Neugarten *et al.*, 1968). Further elaboration of the theory can be found in the previous chapter. Intergenerational programme participation has clearly been viewed as a potential 'new' role for older adults that can contribute towards 'successful ageing' and improved well-being (e.g.

Barton, 1999). This theory and its assumptions support expanding intergenerational programme opportunities to communities throughout North America, Europe and other continents, reaching as many older adults as possible.

By being involved in such programmes, they and the other participants are becoming aware of other generational groups, learn to understand the 'age other' and acquire the ability to sometimes 'give up' their needs to accommodate the needs of other generations – reaching a high Generational Intelligence level. Such a process could enhance social cohesion and social integration.

The terms social cohesion and social integration refer to relationships among different groups of citizens and to the extent to which different groups meet, know, respect and understand each other. The promotion of social cohesion and social integration is therefore aimed at those groups who maintain little or no contact.

Intergenerational programmes provide opportunities for discussing and considering intergenerational differences (real or imagined) at the start of and during the programme. The interest of each discussion lies in new experiences with people from other generations.

The 'social contract' extends the obligations of each member of a society towards the others. As well as a feeling of interdependence, we also need to feel that we belong. In this context, intergenerational programmes are developed with an increased emphasis on goals and outcomes in relation to the concept of 'social inclusion' (Granville and Hatton-Yeo, 2002).

Carefully constructed programmes involve participants in group reflection processes designed to foster critical thinking about how stereotypes tend to weaken the ability to perceive that there are individual differences between people, and that generalizations are never completely accurate (Chamberlain *et al.*, 1994). To sum up, Granville and Hatton-Yeo (2002), for example, point out that intergenerational exchanges can rebuild social networks, develop community capacity and create an inclusive society for all age groups; and Kaplan and Chadha (2004), claim that at the root of intergenerational programmes and practices is a firm belief that we are better off – as individuals, families, communities and as a society – when there are abundant opportunities for young people and older adults to come together to interact, educate, support and otherwise provide care for one another.

Conclusion

In this chapter we viewed the rationale for creating intergenerational community programmes as a method to create 'a society for all ages'. We outlined the development of such programmes, presenting and discussing different types of intergenerational community programmes and their components, analysed the various benefits different groups of participants accrue from these programmes and their contribution at the individual, organizational and community levels. We will finish by analysing how they are an important vehicle on the road for fostering Generational Intelligence.

Clearly, the largest field of research related to intergenerational programmes aims at improving the attitudes of children and adolescents to older persons.

Inter-generational practice helps to increase tolerance, the level of comfort and closeness between young and old, helping to demolish clichés and myths related to the ageing process (Manheimer, 1997). Intergenerational programmes help, thus, to build social cohesion and create an inclusive environment that allows elders to participate fully to the extent of their abilities. The programmes provide purpose while offering a way for people of differing generations to meet, relate and accept each other.

Such programmes present opportunities for participants to place themselves in the position of a person of a different age, or in what has been designated as a different generation. The Generational Intelligence approach is based on the notion of how generations are experienced as part of everyday social life, which happens in various intergenerational programmes. Young and old in such programmes have the opportunity to undergo the four steps outlined in Chapter 1 in order to acquire a high GI: they need to become critically aware of age and generational identity as a factor in social relationships by becoming aware of oneself as being influenced by age and generation, so that they can recognize their personal generational distinctiveness. Following from this is an increased understanding of similarities and differences between generations, becoming critically aware of the values underlying social assumptions about generations and adult ageing and finally, coming to a point where they would act in a manner that will be generationally aware.

Such a process will facilitate an understanding of two key aspects of intergenerational relations. First, the degree to which it is possible to place oneself in the position of the age-other and develop empathy between generations; second, the possibility of working towards negotiated and sustainable solutions. A significant roadblock to the development of empathy towards another generational group, would be forms of social ageism. It was demonstrated in the benefits each of the generations, young and old, obtain from participating in different intergenerational programmes overcoming ageism, and developing a generationally intelligent approach. Such an approach will attempt to make sense of both solidarity and conflict, allowing a relative ability to act with awareness of one's own generational circumstances, while also taking the priorities of other groups into account.

In order to go successfully through this process, it is important to move from an immersive state, where social assumptions about age and generation are taken for granted and the superiority of one's own generational position is assumed; to a more complex state of mind in which multiple perspectives can be recognized, bearing in mind ambiguity and ambivalence; creating intelligent spaces, where conflicting emotions can be contained and links made to members of other groups. We need, though, more evidence of intergenerational programmes contributing to solidarity between adult groups, i.e. people starting families, midlifers, active agers and people who are in deep old age.

Such a view is reflected in The *United Nations Youth Report* (2003) 'One of the central themes running through the Madrid Plan is recognition of the crucial importance of families, intergenerational interdependence, solidarity and reciprocity for social development'. The Plan links the promotion and protection of human rights and fundamental freedoms – including the right to development – to the achievement of '*a society for all ages*' and maybe we should think of '*a society for all generations*'. Again, reciprocity between the generations is emphasized as key. Intergenerational programmes can become a means for building a culture of relationships instead of an individual-oriented culture. The idea is to emphasize a culture involving positive encounters, underlining what happens between people belonging to different generations.

11 Conclusion

Toward sustainable intergenerational relationships

Introduction

Intergenerational relations are in a state of transition that is historically unprecedented. Changing attitudes to adult ageing and perspectives that are largely generationally driven have contributed to a particular form of twenty-first century uncertainty concerning age and intergenerational relationships. Under such conditions, it is easy for resources that are emotional and social in form as well as economic, to appear scarce and act as grounds for conflict as well as fostering protective bonds between members who perceive themselves as belonging to the same group. In response to this historical juncture, we have started a discussion on what has been called Generational Intelligence. The notion of age and generation are closely linked and both are by degrees socially created. What we recognize as age-groups reflect the social construction of divisions based on chronological age and vary from context to context in their salience and boundaries. Similarly, we are placed in generations by historical contexts and shared experiences that are created from outside individuals, who find themselves swept into a series of associations and divisions that shape their experiences of themselves and others. Family, as a marker of lineage, again depends on salience and context to define its influence and its power to direct individual lives. Nevertheless, we argue that the path to negotiating these complex social interactions can begin from increased self-understanding, which frees social actors from their immersive power, and creates the possibility of novel, yet sustainable, critical directions.

As part of this exploration, certain roadblocks to increased Generational Intelligence have been identified. These would include immersion in one's own generational perspective which either excludes or negates alternative perspectives, the simplifying role of binary opposites, the value positions that pre-exist intergenerational relations which generate negative associations based on age or generational division. Stepping beyond these requires the fostering of the relative ability to be aware of one's own prefiguring internal associations, placing oneself in the shoes of the age-other, recognizing the complementary nature of generational differences in building sustainable intergenerational solutions. In order to achieve this, it is necessary to discover places that are both flexible and lasting where critical distance can emerge, creating a space where contradictory thoughts and feelings can be simultaneously held in mind.

Different contexts provoke different degrees of Generational Intelligence and therefore different capacities to evolve and persist over time. In order to find lasting solutions, that respect the dignity of each party, certain steps suggest themselves. These are not simply physical measures, however, but introduce a pathway that starts from a position of uncritical immersion within everyday social stereotypes towards the achievement of a critical space where mixed feelings can be acknowledged and multiple perspectives taken. While in everyday life generation rarely surfaces as a source of personal and social organization, its influence is both deep seated and broad in scope. Generation and age-based identities appear through sustaining a workable sense of self as well as in the structuring of social relations and part of the job of generationally intelligent activity is to make the links between the two. The next link is to reach out to others, who once recognized as distinct, rather than simply extensions of the self, present a challenge that has to be bridged. Here, generationally intelligent activity requires negotiation between generational perspectives and work towards mutually compatible ways of living. If the principal aim of Generational Intelligence is to provide a tool for a deeper understanding of generational relationships and their effects on our everyday lives, the principal objective would be to work towards sustainable generational relations. In this final chapter, we begin a preliminary sketch of what sustainable generational relations might involve.

Sustainable generational relations?

An alignment of identity, emotion and belief between different groups is, according to Thomas *et al.* (2009) an important factor in the development of commitment to sustainable social action. Rather than seeing these alignments as a consequence of solidarity, however, these authors, in a review of the scientific literature, suggest that they can act as pre-requisites and can be fostered to create long-term continuity of action. A common system of meaning is seen as key to ongoing mutual commitment:

> Sustainable identities will be more likely to exist where there is a plausible basis for consensus on relevant issues. . . . Our argument is that sustainable identities require normative consensus about the beliefs and feelings that drive action. . . . a process of crafting a social identity that has a relevant, congruent pattern of norms for action, emotion and efficacy.
>
> (Thomas *et al.*, 2009: 195)

Among the issues that produce such commitment, two stand out in terms of intergenerational relations. The first lies in developing an identity that is oriented towards future change, the second in an emotional identification with others that is closely associated with a strong value stance. When these processes are aligned, they argue, positive collective action takes place.

As Frosh (2003) observes, the urge towards social solidarity has to be addressed in circumstances not of most people's choosing, which somewhat tempers the rush to sustainable relations as 'people are structured by forces over which they do not have control, and that their ongoing engagement with the world is constantly impacted upon by those forces'. However, he goes on to say that it is still possible to retain the power to change those same states of affair, as this: 'is not the same thing as proposing that people have no agency, no capacity to exert influence, or try to understand, resist or rebel' (Frosh, 2003: 1552). Social suffering, arising for example from age prejudice, is according to Frost and Hoggett, 'A reflexive and non-reflexive phenomenon; as something that can be thought about, critically and creatively, and at times is embodied, enacted or projected precisely because it cannot be thought about' (2008: 439). The trick then is to find a way in which emotionally and socially challenging phenomena can move from being unthought to being thought about, while retaining a critical perspective. This, in essence, is what developing generationally intelligent thinking is all about.

In terms of Generational Intelligence, sustainability begins by being mindful of one's own generational circumstances and an ability to empathize with the age-other both emotionally and cognitively. This leads to a series of values and actions that promote negotiated intergenerational relationships. This implies that they must be sustained over time as well as in a shared social space. Taking a number of generational positions into account, finding compromises between different existential positions and interests, taking both past and future relations into account must all be included. Sustainability, in intergenerational terms, means the capacity, as a person, as a social group or as a society, to create generational relationships that last.

Generational present and futures

Wade-Benzoni and Tost have studied intergenerational relations from the perspective of 'intergenerational dilemmas and beneficence'. Taking the example of long-term trends, including global climate change, social insurance systems and national debt, they interrogate the 'trade off between the present and the interests of other people in the future' (2009: 165)

Beneficence refers to 'the extent to which members of present generations are willing to sacrifice their own self interest for the benefit of future others in the absence of economic or material incentives to present actors for doing so' (Wade-Benzoni and Tost, 2009: 166)

A number of studies have indicating that both forms of distance, over space and over time, tend to reduce altruistic and increase self-serving activity (Brennan, 1995; Padilla, 2002; Wade-Benzoni, 2008). However, these authors point out that affinity between current and future generations is, paradoxically, enhanced when first, the future generation has no power to stop or influence current activity (for example, when they are not yet born) and the extent to which 'an individual feels empathetic toward and connected with future others' (Brennan, 1995, p. 171).

Similar trends appear, from other data. People without children will continue to give to younger generations and be more intensely involved in charities and comparable organizations than those with children (Albertini and Kohli, 2009).

Older adults who are subject to potentially contradictory moral discourses such as independence versus social-connectedness, find that these can be managed through an overarching narrative of reciprocity (Breheny and Stephens, 2009). Also, while a number of studies have shown that family reciprocity is likely to depend on the quality of relations across a lifetime (Finch, 1995; Gaalen *et al.*, 2010), and solidarity to be mediated by degree of attachment (Merz *et al.*, 2007), there may be additional factors at play when wider generational beneficence is called for. Wade-Benzoni and Tost argue that when present decision-makers and future generations do not interact, a moral sense of responsibility comes into play making altruistic behaviour more rather than less likely. One driver for future beneficence is reportedly a sense of legacy, which is based on a mix of generativity and desire for immortality 'the desire to invest one's substance in forms of life and work that will outlive the self' (Wade-Benzoni and Tost, 2009: 182). Similarly, emphasizing the beneficent aspects of preceding generation's behaviour can both highlight long-term collective goals and act as a model for current behaviour. The link between identification with past generations and solidarity with future ones is seen to be an important factor here, as well as an ability to identify with them. This is especially true when current generations are encouraged to put themselves in the place of future ones and ask themselves how they would like to have been treated by preceding generations themselves. Such acts of reciprocal empathic understanding chime well with increased Generational Intelligence, but include a serious omission:

> Generation, used in the sense of 'future generations', holds a certain disadvantage in terms of our own definition of generational sustainability, as this form of inquiry assumes that while the interests of current decision-makers may be in conflict with future others 'there is no opportunity for future generations to directly reciprocate the good or bad given to them by prior generations'
>
> (Wade-Benzoni and Tost, 2009: 166)

In other words the generations in question are seen not to overlap, thus precluding direct interaction though a combination of both interpersonal and temporal distance. Thus, the discourse on generational beneficence primarily addresses empathy from older to younger ages, and does not explore the relationship from younger to older. It also fails to explore how coexisting generations might interact and find ways of living together. In so doing, it omits the ways that contemporary generational relations influence future planning.

A further limitation of beneficence research is that, in limiting its definition of generational exchange, it rarely takes wider inequities into account, and does not consider the effects of other forms of re-distribution on intergenerational relations. The effect of more unequal market systems on interpersonal relationships can, according to Bauman (2003), be that relationships are only entered 'for what can be derived by each person' and 'continued only in so far as it is thought by both parties to deliver enough satisfaction for each individual to stay with it' (2003: 89). Further, economically egalitarian systems appear to provide a greater sense of citizen well-being and reciprocity than those that foster greater inequality between wealth and income (Wilkinson and Pickett, 2009; Andersen *et al.*, 2007). Wilkinson and Pickett (2009) show this across an impressive number of quality indicators such as life expectancy, infant mortality, crime rates, literacy scores and even degree of re-cycling. It is, in other words, the size of the gap between the top and bottom 20 per cent of the population that influences general well-being rather than overall national wealth and gross domestic product. Societies with large differences, such as the US and the UK tend to rely on fear of failure as a mechanism rather than social solidar-ity, even though this increases social stress for all members. Andersen *et al.* (2007) argue that the Nordic social model, which embraces globalization and shares risk across social groups has maintained both economic competitiveness and a strong sense of social cohesion, leading to higher levels of well-being. As pensions, health care and older workers are increasingly becoming issues of social solidarity, the relationship between socio-economic context and intergenerational relations should not be so easily ignored.

If Freud was right and the suppression of self-interest is the defining characteris-tic of civilized life, then it raises a question about what should be done with social models that foster intergenerational competition. These models tend to focus on exchanges in the here and now, with little emphasis on future consequences or past commitments. And as Frosh (2003) has pointed out, such social conditions drive a wedge between self and others. A counterweight to these tendencies that atom-ize relationships and strip them back to immediate instrumental advantage, lies in the capacity to place oneself in the position of the other and to locate sources of solidarity, that make for lasting and positive social relations. In this case, between generations.

Building sustainable intergenerational relationships

We would argue that sustainable intergenerational relationships will need to rely on increased levels of insight, empathy and mutually negotiated action and that these are more likely to emerge in social situations that foster forms of generational coopera-tion rather than competition. Intelligence of this sort facilitates the interplay between different levels of understanding associated with intergenerational exchanges. Ulti-mately, such deeper understanding should allow us to move beyond binary concep-tual positions, such as macro or micro, present or future, profit or loss, which can so often give credence to inflexible responses to related social dilemmas. An intelligent approach to intergenerational relations would need to address the issue of how indi-viduals become self-consciously aware of their generational status and how far it influences their experience of and action towards sustainable generational relations. Some of these have been sketched out in this book, including the creation of critical space via masquerade and a shift from binary opposition to the tolerance of ambiva-lence and ambiguity.

While the content of sustainable solutions in specified areas would be difficult to determine in advance, it may be possible to outline what a generally high or low generationally intelligent response might be like. Sustainability in this context would rely on solutions that will endure, where the costs to parties are not too great and are balanced by compatible activities and where tensions, in feeling, thinking and doing, can be contained in a viable phenomenal space.

Biggs and Lowenstein (2010) identified different elements of Generational Intelligence that would contribute to high and low states of generationally sustainable solutions. Each element reflects one of the contributions to generational phenomenology which, when recombined would build towards a novel process of understanding inter-generational relations and the ability to engage empathically with the age-other over time. Starting from the personal life course, a high level of Generational Intelligence offers an insight that people develop and change with particular priorities that arise as their own life progresses. To which can be added acknowledgement that family roles change according to age and position in the family, the degree of interdependence of generations at any one time, an understanding of which enhances communication and shared problem-solving. Further, being aware of one's own cohort membership or the salience of cohort for participating generations, may facilitate balancing the demands of different cohort groups. Taken together, insight into one's own position (in the life course), an understanding of generationally inflected relationships to others (in families or at work) and an understanding of the power of the social context in which relations take place (through cohort membership or particular policy arenas), increases the likelihood of generationally intelligent solutions emerging.

At a personal level, low levels of Generational Intelligence would be reflected in an immersion in one's position, either by acting exclusively in the present, asserting the primacy of that position without taking other ones into account, splitting off or rejecting ambivalent feelings. One's personal phenomenology is presumed to be universally valid. In terms of family relations, there would be an unwillingness or lack of interest to reflect upon or recognize complex relationships between social actors, resulting in low-quality exchange relations marked by a lack of reciprocity. In terms of cohort culture, an assumption that one's own age group is dominant leads to positions where generations are perceived to be essentially the same, or irrelevant to dominant interests. Thus a low level of Generational Intelligence fails to travel beyond its own cohort experience, showing little interest in alternative perspectives. Generally speaking, a low generationally intelligent phenomenology would be unable to reflect on its own position and thereby engage in sustainable temporal relationships. Immersion in simple unreflective experience results in a failure to distinguish between life course, family and cohort influences, and an inability to move beyond simple assimilation of the age-other into that static perspective.

Negotiating generational sustainability

How, then, can a sense of the specialness of each part of the adult life course be established, and the likelihood of harmony, rather than competition be fostered between generational groups over time?

It may be premature to specify the contents of such a sustainable settlement. It would depend upon the expression of existential priorities that adults have been encouraged, culturally speaking, to suppress. It will take time to get beyond the socially correct answers of wanting to work longer, claiming that one does not grow old and that there are effectively no generational differences that pervade advanced economies. Generationally intelligent work would head towards the creation of spaces that foster the discovery of alternative pathways and of pluralistic, yet more subversive discourses.

Part of the answer might lie in finding ways of balancing intergenerational priorities. Rather than trying to be the same regardless of age, we should perhaps attempt a course that explores complementary role relations based on the recognition of generational distinctiveness. The point here is that without basing intergenerational negotiation on the recognition of substantive differences as well as commonalities, any solutions are unlikely to stand the test of time. They are in this sense unsustainable. In order to ground negotiation, the series of assumptive realities outlined earlier in this book would need to be set aside, so that they can be seen with the benefit of critical distance rather than through cultural immersion. Space for sustainable cultural growth is thereby created.

To achieve this, in process terms, it might be worth briefly re-visiting the steps towards Generational Intelligence outlined by Biggs, Haapala and Lowenstein (2011) and elaborated at the beginning of this book.

The first of these would be for social actors to critically locate themselves within a distinguishable generational group. This would help to clarify the specific existential tasks, associated with a particular part of the life course. It would involve a process of self-reflection as well as the establishment of a complex rather than an immersive relationship with contemporary social expectations.

The second would be to increase explicit awareness of generational distinctiveness and the balance between difference and similarity of interest. This would avoid the trap of thinking that all age groups hold essentially the same priorities and needs. It would include a process of separation and return from the age-other in order to establish evolution over time and a connection that recognizes the age-other as more than an extension of one's own priorities.

The third includes making a value judgement in terms of one's position on the quality of this differential relationship, in terms of conflict and cooperation, holding potentially contradictory elements in mind without succumbing to oppositional thinking. In terms of increased Generational Intelligence, this stage would include the development of a-symmetrical complementarity.

Finally action would be considered, based on intergenerational negotiation. Such negotiation would need to be mindful of the opportunities for recognizing distinctiveness while at the same time discovering areas of common cause. It would begin from the position that the projects of different generational groups are equally valid, yet accommodation towards sustainable solutions requires compromise.

According to this model, existing policy initiatives such as an investment in longevity research and in work-based productive ageing may be missing some important factors in the management of adult ageing and intergenerational relationships. Most notably, there are differences between generations in terms of their life tasks and existential positions which are culturally eclipsed, yet vital to an enriched and age-inclusive society. Such a statement would not be necessary were it not for the fact that people so often take age and generation for granted. So that, while we all too often act on the basis of stereotypical judgements, we assume these are unremarkable. They nevertheless exist in the context of imbalances of power at a number of levels, in terms of personal identity, interpersonally, inter-group and structural allocation of resources. These assumptions help to explain why putting oneself in the shoes of the age-other appears so easy. Essentially, when we think we are seeing something from the perspective of the age-other we are making a life-course category error. A mistake that is based primarily on the dominance of younger adulthood and midlife priorities, backed up by economic considerations grafted onto population ageing from other domains. In order to re-discover a more authentic purpose for a long life, it is necessary to create critical distance from these assumptive realities, and it is here that Generational Intelligence might be of some service.

Strategies, values and generational intelligent action

Under such conditions, identity needs to be negotiated, and circumstances will vary depending on the degree of generational expression they afford. There will be a need to both protect identity and connect with the wider social world, through forms of impression management and masquerade. In the process the self becomes layered, with some aspects finding expression and others having to be put aside in the interests of negotiated compromise. Thinking about the maintenance of intergenerational relations in this way raises a number of interesting questions for a generationally intelligent agency. First, any tension between connection and separateness would need to find the optimum level for both. We all need contact with other people, even if that contact is sometimes disconfirming and causes us to withdraw. Overcoming age-dominance would form one important constituent of that context. The expression of intergenerational solidarity and the likelihood that the internal world can be expressed in any one external space would contribute to the identification of sustainable intergenerational solutions. It would allow us to ask whether particular policies facilitate or inhibit the expression of cohesive generational relations. Where the likelihood is greater, so would the possibilities for more genuine self-expression and liberating negotiation. Finally, these obser-vations free us from recourse to particular content in identifying negative relations rather, degrees of Generational Intelligence provide a conceptual tool for inter-rogating the spaces that policy might create for sustainable generational relation-ships. As narratives of ageing change, legitimized forms of interaction also change. However, this says little in itself about the appropriateness of these narratives for ageing or for sustainability and to address this problem, we must also return to the question of complexity. An analysis taking complexity into account would ask whether it is enough that available spaces provide admission into a world marked by social conformity. This would only force generational relations back into an interior space, where aspects of the self that are not allowed legitimate expression can exist consciously, or unconsciously and raises questions about what happens to relations that are beyond the limitations set by legitimizing social narratives. In any novel policy context, it should be asked, what will surface and what will be hidden in the new narrative that emerges, and thus what will become conforming and what subversive.

In this book, we have only really made a tentative first step towards understanding intergenerational relations between adults. Our examples have largely been restricted and incomplete. However, we believe that examining degrees of Generational Intelligence and discovering the contexts in which it can be increased is a worthwhile enterprise, which can be undertaken as a journey of self-exploration, of social interaction and in the service of more developed policies for a changing intergenerational world.

Bibliography

AARP (2007). *AARP Profit From Experience*. (AARP) September 2007. http://assets.aarp. org/rgcenter/econ/intl_older_worker.pdf (Retrieved 5/5/08).

AARP Report (2008). *Valuing the Invaluable: The Economic Value of Family Caregiving*. Washington, US: AARP Public Policy Institute.

Aboderin, I. (2004). Modernization and ageing theory revisited: Current explanations of recent developing world and historical Western shifts in material family support for older people. *Ageing and Society*, 24(1), 29–50.

Action on Elder Abuse (2010). http://www.elderabuse.org.uk/ (Retrieved 10/3/10).

Aday, R.H., McDuffie, W. and Sims, C.R. (1993). Impact of an intergenerational program on Black adolescents' attitudes toward the elderly. *Educational Gerontology*, 19, 663–73.

Adler, R.P. (2003). *The Potential of Older Workers for Staffing California's After-School Programs*. San Francisco: Civic Ventures.

Agree, E., Bissett, B. and Rendall, M. (2003). Simultaneous care for parents and care for children among mid-life British women. *Population Trends*, 112(1), 29–35.

Alber, J. and Kohler, U. (2004). *Health and Care in an Enlarged Europe*. European Foundation for the Improvement of Living and Working Conditions. Luxembourg: Office for Official Publications of the European Communities.

Albertini, M. and Kohli, M. (2009). What childless older people give: Is the generational link broken? *Ageing and Society*, 29(4), 1261–74.

Albertini, M., Kohli, M. and Vogel, C. (2007). Intergenerational transfers of time and money in European families: Common patterns – different regimes? *Journal of European Social Policy*, 17(4), 319–34.

Andersen, T.M., Holmstrom, B. and Honkapohja, S. (2007). *The Nordic Model: Embracing Globalisation and Sharing Risks*. Helsinki: ETLA, 164.

Andrews, F.M. (1986). *Research on the Quality of Life*. Institute for Social Research, University of Michigan: Ann Arbor.

Andrews, F.M. and Withey, S.B. (1976). *Social Indicators of Well-Being: American Perceptions of Life Quality*. New York: Plenum.

Aneshensel, C.S., Pearlin, L.I., Mullan, J.T., Zarit, S.H. and Whitlatch, C.J. (1995). *Profiles in Caregiving. The Unexpected Career*. San Diego: Academic Press.

Antonucci, T.C., Akiyama, H. and Merline, A. (2001). Dynamics of social relationships in midlife. In M. E. Lachman (Ed.), *Handbook of Midlife Development* (pp. 571–98). New York: Wiley.

Antonucci, T.C., Jackson, J.S. and Biggs, S. (2007). Intergenerational relations: Theory, research, and policy. *Journal of Social Issues*, 63(4), 679–93.

Arber, S. and Attias-Donfut, C. (2000). *The Myth of Generational Conflict*. London: Routledge.

Arno, P.S. (2002). *Economic Value of Informal Caregiving*. Paper presented at the American Association for Geriatric Psychiatry Orlando, Florida, February 24, 2002.

Atchley, R.C. (1972). Retirement. *The Gerontologist*, 12(4), 436–40.

Atchley, R.C. (1989). A continuity theory of normal aging. *The Gerontologist*, 29(2), 183–90.

Atkinson, M.P., Kivett, V.R. and Campbell, R.T. (1986). Intergenerational solidarity: An examination of a theoretical model. *Journal of Gerontology*, 41(3), 408–13.

Attias-Donfut, C. (1988). *Sociologie des Générations: L'empreinte du Temps*. Paris, Puf.

Attias-Donfut, C. (2000). Cultural and economic transfers between generations: One aspect of age integration. *The Gerontologist*, 40, 270–72.

Attias-Donfut, C. (2003). Family transfers and cultural transmissions between three generations in France. In V.L. Bengtson and A. Lowenstein (Eds), *Global Aging and Challenges to Families* (pp. 214–52). New York: Aldine de Gruyter.

Attias-Donfut, C. (2005). *Transferencias Intrafamiliares y Dinámicas Sociales*. Viejas sociedades, nueva – Centro de Investigaciones.

Attias-Donfut, C. (2007). *The Three Generations' Survey – Measuring Family Support in Europe*. CNAV, FRANCE – Southern Universities Press.

Attias-Donfut, C. and Wolff, F.C. (2005). Generational memory and family relationships. In M.L. Johnson (Ed.), *The Cambridge Handbook of Age and Ageing* (443–54). Cambridge: Cambridge University Press.

Attias-Donfut, C., Ogg, J. and Wolff, F. (2005). European patterns of intergenerational financial and time transfers. *European Journal of Ageing*, 2, 161–73.

Bales, S.S., Eklund, S.J. and Siffin, C.F. (2000). Children's perceptions of elders before and after a school-based intergenerational program. *Educational Gerontology*, 26, 677–89.

Ballard, K., Elston, M. and Gabe, J. (2005). Beyond the mask: Experiences of public and private ageing during midlife and their use in age-resisting activities. *Health*, 9(2), 169–87.

Baltes, P.B. and Baltes, M.M. (1990). Psychological perspectives on successful aging: The model of selective optimization with compensation. In P.B. Baltes and M.M. Baltes (Eds), *Successful Aging: Perspectives from the Behavioral Sciences* (pp. 1–34). New York: Cambridge University Press.

Baltes, P.B., Freund, A.M. and Li, S.C. (2005). The psychological science of human ageing. In M.L. Johnson (Ed.), *The Cambridge Handbook of Age and Ageing* (pp. 67–71). Cambridge, England: Cambridge University Press.

Banerjee, A., Daly, T., Armstrong, H., Lafrance, S. and Szebehely, M. (2008). *Out of Control: Violence Against Support Workers in Long Term Care*. York: Canada: York University Press.

Barton, H. (1999). Effects of an intergenerational program on the attitudes of emotionally disturbed youth toward the elderly. *Educational Gerontology*, 25, 623–40.

Bauman, Z. (1991). Modernity and ambivalence. *Theory, Culture and Society*, 7, 143–69.

Bauman, Z. (1995). *Life in Fragments: Essays in Postmodern Morality*. Oxford: Blackwell.

Bauman, Z. (1997). *Postmodernity and its Discontents*. New York: New York University Press.

Bauman, Z. (2003). *Liquid Love: On the Frailty of Human Bonds*. Cambridge: Polity Press.

Bauman, Z. (2004). *Wasted Lives: Modernity and its Outcasts*. London: Polity Press.

Bengtson, V.L. (1993). Is the 'contract across generations' changing? Effects of population aging on obligations and expectations across age groups. In V.L. Bengtson and W.A. Achenbaum (Eds), *The Changing Contract Across Generations* (pp. 3–23). New York: Aldine de Gruyter.

Bengtson, V.L. (2001). The Burgess Award Lecture: Beyond the nuclear family: The increasing importance of multigenerational bonds. *Journal of Marriage and the Family*, 63(1), 1–16.

Bengtson, V.L. and Lowenstein, A. (2003). *Global Aging and Challenges to Families*. New York: Aldine de Gruyter.

Bengtson, V.L. and Murray, T.M. (1993). Justice across generations (and cohorts): Sociological perspectives on the life course and reciprocities over time. In L.M. Cohen (Ed.), *Justice Across Generations: What Does it Mean?* (pp. 11–138). Washington, DC: AARP.

Bengtson, V.L. and Putney, N.M. (2006). Future 'conflicts' across generations and cohorts? In J. Vincent, C. Phillipson and M. Downs (Eds), *The Futures of Old Age* (pp. 20–29). London: Sage.

Bengtson, V.L. and Roberts, R.E. (1991). Intergenerational solidarity in aging families: An example of formal theory construction. *Journal of Marriage and the Family*, 53, 856–70.

Bengtson, V.L. and Schrader, S. (1982). Parent-child relations. In D. Mangen and W. A. Peterson (Eds), *Research Instruments in Social Gerontology* (Vol. 2, pp. 115–86). Minneapolis: University of Minnesota Press.

Bengtson, V.L., Elder, G.H. and Putney, N.M. (2005). The lifecourse perspective on ageing: Linked lives, timing, and history. In M.L. Johnson (Ed.), *The Cambridge Handbook of Age and Ageing* (pp. 493–501). Cambridge: Cambridge University Press.

Bengtson, V.L., Rosenthal, C. and Burton, L. (1990). Families and aging: Diversity and heterogeneity. In R.H. Binstock and L.K. George (Eds), *Handbook of Aging and the Social Sciences* (3rd ed., pp. 263–87). San Diego, CA: Academic Press.

Bengtson, V.L., Schaie, K.W. and Burton, L.M. (Eds) (1995). *Adult Intergenerational Relations: Effects of Societal Change*. New York: Springer.

Bengtson, V.L., Giarrusso, R., Mabry, J. and Silverstein, M. (2002). Solidarity, conflict and ambivalence: Complementary or competing perspectives on intergenerational relationships? *Journal of Marriage and Family*, 64(3), 568–76.

Bengtson, V.L., Giarrusso, R., Silverstein, M. and Wang, H. (2000). Families and intergenerational relationships in aging societies. *Hallym International Journal of Aging*, 2(1), 3–10.

Bengtson, V.L., Lowenstein, A., Putney, N.M. and Gans, D. (2003). Global aging and the challenges to families. In V.L. Bengtson and A. Lowenstein (Eds), *Global Aging and Challenges to Families* (pp. 1–26). New York: Aldine de Gruyter.

Bengtson, V.L., Acock, A.C., Allen, K.A., Dilworth-Anderson, P. and Klein, D.M. (2005). Theory and theorizing in family research. In V.L. Bengtson, A.C. Acock, K.R. Allen, P. Dilworth-Andersen and D.M. Klein (Eds), *Sourcebook on Family Theory and Research* (pp. 3–33). New York: Sage Publications.

Berger, D.M. (1987). *Clinical Empathy*. Northvale: Jason Aronson, Inc.

Berger, P. and Luckman, T. (1966). *The Social Construction of Reality: A Treatise in the Sociology of Knowledge*. Garden City, NY: Doubleday

Berger, P. and Luckman, T. (1976). *The Social Construction of Reality*. London: Penguin.

Bergstrom, M.J. and Holmes, M.E. (2000). Lay theories of successful aging after the death of a spouse: A network text analysis of bereavement advice. *Health Communication*, 12(4), 377–406.

Berkman, L.F. and Kawachi, I. (2000). *Social Epidemiology*. New York: Oxford University Press.

Bernard, M., Bartlam, B., Simm, J. and Biggs, S. (2007). Housing and care for older people: Life in an English purpose built retirement village. *Ageing and Society*, 27(4), 555–78.

Bernard, M., Biggs, S., Bartlam, B. and Sim, J. (2004). *New Lifestyles in Old Age: Health, Identity and Wellbeing in Retirement Communities*. Bristol: Policy Press.

Biggs, S. (1989). Professional resistances to work with older people. *Ageing and Society*, 9, 43–60.

Biggs, S. (1992). Attitudes, ageing and group work. In K. Morgan (Ed.), *Responding to an Ageing Society* (pp. 84–98). Chichester: J. Wiley.

Biggs, S. (1993). Interprofessional collaboration and user participation. *Journal of Interprofessional Care*, 7(2), 151–59.

Biggs, S. (1999). *The Mature Imagination: Dynamics of Identity in Mid-Life and Beyond*. Bucks: Open University Press.

Biggs, S. (2001). Toward critical narrativity: Stories of aging in contemporary social policy. *Journal of Aging Studies*, 15(4), 303–16.

Biggs, S. (2004). Narratives, masquerades, feminism and gerontology. *Journal of Ageing Studies*, 18(1), 45–58.

Biggs, S. (2005). Beyond appearances: Perspectives on identity in later life and some implications for method. *Journal of Gerontology: Social Sciences*, 69B, S118–27.

Biggs, S. (2006). Ageing selves and others: Distinctiveness and uniformity in the struggle for intergenerational solidarity. In J. A. Vincent, C. Phillipson and M. Downs (Eds), *The Futures of Old Age* (Chapter 10, p. 115). London: Sage.

Biggs, S. (2007). Thinking about generations: Conceptual positions and policy implications. *Journal of Social Issues*, 63(4), 695–712.

Biggs, S. (2008). Facing Retirement Forum: Leading the Debate. *Commentary on Second Wave Data of the International Retirement Index*. London: The Hartford.

Biggs, S. and Lowenstein, A. (forthcoming). Toward Generational Intelligence: Linking cohorts, families and experience. In M. Silverstein and R. Giarousso (Eds), *From Generation to Generation: Continuity and Change in Aging Families*. The Johns Hopkins University Press.

Biggs, S., Haapala, I. and Lowenstein, A. (2011) Exploring generational intelligence as a model for examining the process of intergenerational relationships. *Ageing and Society*, 31(1), 1–18.

Biggs, S., Lowenstein, A. and Hendricks, J. (2003). *The Need for Theory: Critical Approaches to Social Gerontology*. Amityville, NY: Baywood Publishing Co. Inc.

Biggs, S., Bernard, M., Kingston, P. and Nettleton, H. (2000). Lifestyles of belief: Narrative and culture in a retirement community. *Ageing and Society* 20(6), 649–72.

Biggs, S., Phillipson, C., Money, A.M. and Leach, R. (2006). The age shift: Observations on social policy, ageism and the dynamics of the adult lifecourse. *Journal of Social Work Practice*, 20(3), 239–50

Biggs, S., Phillipson, C., Money, A.M. and Leach, R. (2007). The mature imagination and consumption strategies: Age and generation in the development of baby boomer identity. *International Journal of Ageing and Later Life*, 2(2), 31–59.

Biggs, S., Stevens, M., Tinker, A., Dixon. J. and Lee, L. (2010). Institutional Mistreatment and Dignity, toward a conceptual understanding. NATCEN Research Paper. NATCEN, London.

Biggs, S., McCreadie, C., Manthorpe, J., Tinker, A., Hills, A., Doyle, M. and Erens, B. (2009). Mistreatment of older people in the United Kingdom: Findings from the first national prevalence study. *Journal of Elder Abuse and Neglect*, 21(1), 1–14.

Billing, M., Condor, S., Edwards, D., Gane, M., Middleton, D. and Radley, A. (1988). *Ideological Dilemmas*. Beverly Hills: Sage Publications.

Blumer, H. (1971). Social problems as collective behaviour. *Social Problems*, 18(3), 298–306.

Bollas, C. (1987). *The Shadow of the Object*. London: Free Association Books.

Bollas, C. (1992). *Being a Character: Psychoanalysis and Self-Experience*. London: Free Association Press.

Bonnie, R.J. and Wallace, R.B. (2003). *Elder Mistreatment: Abuse, Neglect and Exploitation in an Aging America*. Washington DC: National Research Council.

Bourdieu, P. (1979). *La Distinction: Critique Social du Jugement*. Paris: Editions de minuit.

Bourdieu, P. (1996). On the family as a realized category. *Theory, Culture and Society*, 13(3), 19–26.

Bowling, A. (1993). The concept of successful and positive aging, *Family Practice*, 10(4), 449–53.

Bowling, A. (2005). *Ageing Well: Quality of Life in Old Age*. Berkshire: England, Open University Press.

Bowling, A. (2007). Aspirations for older age in the 21st century: What is successful aging? *The International Journal of Aging and Human Development*, 64(3), 263–97.

Bowling, A. and Dieppe, P. (2005). What is successful aging and who should define it? *British Medical Journal*, 331, 1548–551.

Bowling, A., See-Tai, S., Shah, E., Gabriel, Z. and Solanki, P. (2005). Attribute of age identity. *Aging and Society*, 25(4), 479–500.

Brammer, A. (2006). Domestic violence crime and victims act 2004. *Journal of Adult Protection*, 8(1), 50–53.

Brandtstädter, J. and Rothermund, K. (2002). The life-course dynamics of goal pursuit and goal adjustment: A two-process framework. *Developmental Review*, 22(1), 117–50.

Breheny, M. and Stephens, C. (2009). 'I sort of pay back in my own little way': Managing independence and social connectedness through reciprocity. *Ageing and Society*, 29(8), 1295–1313.

Brennan, T.J. (1995). Discounting the future: Economics and ethics. *Resources*, 120, 3–6.

Brody, E.M. (1981). Women in the middle and family help to older people. *The Gerontologist*, 21(5), 471–80.

Brodsky, J., Habib, J., Hirschfeld, M. and Siegel, B. (2002). Care of the frail elderly in developed and developing countries: The experience and the challenges. *Aging: Clinical and Experimental Research*, 14(4), 279–86.

Bronfenbrenner, U. (1979). *The Ecology of Human Development: Experiments by Nature and Design*. Cambridge, MA: Harvard University Press.

Brooke, R. (1991). *Jung and Phenomenology*. London: Routledge

Butler, R.N. (1975). *Why Survive? Being Old in America*. Harper and Row: New York.

Butler, R.N. (1987). Ageism. In G.L. Maddox and R.C. Atchley (Eds), *The Encyclopedia of Aging* (pp. 22–23). New York: Springer.

Butler, R.N. (1989). Dispelling ageism: The cross-cutting intervention. *Annals of the American Academy of Political and Social Sciences*, 503, 138–47.

Butler, R.N. and Gleason, H.P. (1985). *Productive Aging*. New York: Springer.

Butler, R.N. and Schechter, M. (1995). Productive Aging. In G. Maddox, *The Encyclopaedia of Aging*. New York: Springer.

Butler, R.N., Miller, R.A., Perry, D., Carnes, B.A., Williams, T.F., Cassel, C., Brody, J., Bernard, M.A., Partridge, L., Kirkwood, T., Martin, G.M. and Olshansky, S.J. (2008). New model of health promotion and disease prevention for the 21st century. *British Medical Journal*, 337, 337–99

Bytheway, B. (1994). *Ageism*. Buckingham: Open University Press.

Bytheway, B. (2005). Ageism. In M.L. Johnson, V.L. Bengtson, P.G. Coleman and T.B.L. Kirkwood (Eds), *The Cambridge Handbook on Age and Ageing* (pp. 338–46). Cambridge: Cambridge University Press.

Cain, L.D. Jr. (1964). Life course and social structure. In R.E.L. Faris (Ed.), *Handbook of Modern Sociology* (pp. 272–309). Chicago: Rand Mcnally.

Calasanti, T. (2003). Masculinities and care work in old age. In S. Arber, K. Davidson and J. Ginn (Eds), *Gender and Aging: Changing Roles and Relationships* (pp. 15–30). Maidenhead, UK: Open University Press.

Campbell, A., Converse, P. and Rogers, W. (1976). *The Quality of American Life*. New York: Russell Sage Foundation.

Cantor, M.H. (1975). Life space and the social support systems of the inner city elderly of New York. *Gerontologist*, 15(1), 23–27.

Cantor, M.H. (1980). The informal support system: Its relevance in the lives of the elderly. In E.F. Borgatta and N. McClusky (Eds), *Aging and Society* (pp. 47–54). Beverly Hills, CA: Sage.

Caro, F., Bass, S., and Chen, Y. (1993). *Achieving a Productive Aging Society*. Westport: Auburn House.

Carstensen, L.L. (1995). Evidence for a life-span theory of socioemotional selectivity. *Current Directions in Psychological Science*, 4, 151–56.

Chamberlain, V.M., Fetterman, E. and Maher, M. (1994). Innovation in elder and child care: An intergenerational experience. *Educational Gerontology*, 19, 193–204.

Chamie, J. (2010). Population Aging: A Human Triumph. *Globalist*. http://www.theglobal-ist.com/StoryId.aspx?StoryId = 8577 (Retrieved 12/7/10).

Chauvel, L. (2007a). *Les Nouvelles Générations Devant la Panne Prolongée de L'ascenseur Social*, Source internet, http://louis.chauvel.free.fr/ofceralentissementgenerationnel5. pdf (consulté le 7.11.2007).

Chauvel, L. (2007b). Social generations, life chances and welfare regime sustainability. In D. Pepper (Ed.), *Changing France: The Politics That Markets Make*. New York: Palgrave MacMillan.

Cheren, L. (2000). *Life's Work: Generational Attitudes Toward Work and Life Integration*. Conducted by the Radcliffe Public Policy Center with Harris Interactive, Inc. Sponsored by FleetBoston Financial.

Childs, H.W., Hayslip Jr., B., Radika, L.M. and Reinberg, J.A. (2000). Young and middle aged adults' perceptions of elder abuse. *The Gerontologist*, 40(1), 75–85.

Chodorow, J. (1997). *Jung on Active Imagination*. London: Routledge.

Cicirelli, V. (2003). Mothers' and daughters' paternalism beliefs and caregiving decision making. *Research on Aging*, 25(1), 3–21.

Civic Ventures (2001). *Recasting Retirement* (p. 4). San Francisco.

Civic Ventures (2005). *Appealing to Experience* (pp. 24–25). San Francisco.

Civil Service (2000). *Winning the Generation Game*. CABI 99–5267/004/D16. London: Civil Service.

Clain, O. (2005). The baby boomer generation and ideologies in Quebec. *Vital Aging*, 11(2), 4–5.

Clark, R.L. and Quinn, J.F. (2002). Patterns of work and retirement for a new century. *Generations*, 26(2), 17–24.

Clarke, L.H. and Griffin, M. (2007). The body natural and the body unnatural: Beauty work and aging. *Journal of Aging Studies*, 21(3), 187–201.

Collard, D. (2001). The generational bargain. *Intergenerational Journal of Social Welfare*, 10(1), 54–65.

Connidis, I.A. (2001). *Family Ties and Aging.* Thousand Oaks, CA: Sage.

Connidis, I.A. and McMullin, J.A. (2002a). Ambivalence, family ties, and doing sociology. *Journal of Marriage and Family*, 64(3), 594–601.

Connidis, I.A. and McMullin, J.A. (2002b). Sociological ambivalence and family ties: A critical perspective. *Journal of Marriage and Family*, 64(3), 558–67.

Cook Ross Inc. (2004). *Managing a Multigenerational Workforce: The Diversity Managers Toolkit.* http://www.thediversitytoolkit.com/managers/pdfs/Managing%20a%20Multige nerational%20Workforce.pdf (Retrieved 28/5/08).

Cook, F.L. and Barrett, E.J. (1992). *Support for the American Welfare State.* New York: Columbia University Press.

Cooper, C., Selwood, A., Blanchard, M., Walker, Z., Blizard, R. and Livingston, G. (2009). Abuse of people with dementia by family carers: Representative cross sectional survey. *British Medical Journal*, 338(b), 155–57.

Corsten, M. (1999). The time of generations. *Time and Society*, 8(2), 249–72.

Coupland, N. (2004). Age in social and sociolinguistic theory. In J. Nussbaum and J. Coupland (Eds), *Handbook of Communication and Aging Research* (pp. 69–90). Mahwah, New Jersey.

Coupland, J. (2009). Time, the body and the reversibility of ageing. *Ageing and Society*, 29: Special Issue 06: 953–76.

Craib, I. (2001). *Psychoanalysis: A Critical Introduction.* Cambridge: Polity.

Daatland, S.O. (2008). How to balance generations: Solidarity dilemmas in a European perspective. In R. Edmondson and H.-J. von Kondratowitz (Eds), *Valuing Older People: A Humanist Approach to Ageing* (pp. 123–38). Bristol: Policy Press.

Daatland, S.O. and Herlofson, K. (2003). 'Lost solidarity' or 'changed solidarity': A comparative European view of normative family solidarity. *Ageing and Society*, 23(5), 537–60.

Daatland, S.O. and Lowenstein, A. (2005). Intergenerational solidarity and the family–welfare state balance. *European Journal of Aging*, 2(3), 174–82.

Daatland, S.O., Herlofson, K. and Lima, I.A. (2010). Balancing generations: On the strength and character of family norms in the West and East of Europe. *Norwegian Social Research (NOVA)*, Oslo Norway.

Daly, C. and Jogerst, A. (2006). Definitions in nursing home statutes USA. *Journal of Elder Abuse and Neglect*, 18(1), 23–29.

Dannefer, D. (2008). New twists in the paths of the life course. In V. Bengtson, M. Silverstein and N. Putney (Eds), *Handbook of Theories of Aging.* New York: Springer (with Jessica Kelley-Moore).

Davey, A. and Szinovacz, M.E. (2008). Division of care among adult children. In A. Davey and M.E. Szinovacz (Eds), *Caregiving Contexts: Cultural, Familial and Societal Implications* (pp. 133–59). New York: Springer Publishing Co.

De Beauvoir, S. (1970). *Old Age.* London: Penguin.

De Jong Gierveld, J., Dykstra, P.A. and Schenk, N. (2009). *Living Arrangements and Differences in Family Support: A Comparative Perspective.* Seminar on Family Support Networks and Population Aging, Doha, Qatar, 3–4 June 2009.

Dearden, C. and Becker, S. (2004). *Young Carers in the United Kingdom: The 2004 Report*. Leicestershire, England: Loughborough University.

Demakakos, P., Hacker, E. and Gjonca, E. (2005). Perceptions of ageing. In *The English Longitudinal Study of Ageing Report*. Chapter 11 (p. 14). London: ELSA.

Den Dulk, L. (2005). Workplace work-family arrangements: A study and explanatory framework of differences between organizational provisions in different welfare states. In S. Poelmans (Ed.), *Work and Family: An International Research Perspective* (pp. 211–38). Mahwah, NJ: Lawrence Erlbaum Associates.

Department of Health (1993). *No Longer Afraid*. London: HMSO.

Department of Health (2000). *No Secrets*. London: Department of Health.

Department of Health. (2008). *Safeguarding Adults: A Consultation*. London: Department of Health.

Dittmann-Kohli, F. (1990). Sinngebung im Alter. In P. Mayring and W. Saup (Eds), *Entwicklungs-prozesse im Alter* (pp. 145–66). Stuttgart, Berlin, Köln: Kohlhammer.

Dittmann-Kohli, F. (2005). Self and identity. In M. Johnson (Ed.), *The Cambridge Handbook of Age and Ageing* (pp. 275–91). Cambridge: Cambridge University Press.

Dittmann-Kohli, F. and Joop, D. (2007). Self and life management. In J. Bond, S. Peace, F. Dittmann-Kohli and G. Westerhoff (Eds), *Ageing in Society* (pp. 268–95). London: Sage.

Dobbs, J., Healey, P., Kane, K., Mak, D. and McNamara, T. (2007). *The Multi-Generational Workplace*. Fact Sheet 09, The Center on Aging and Work/Workplace Flexibility at Boston College. Available at www.bc.edu/agingandwork (Retrieved 9/12/09).

Dobson, A. (2000). *Green Political Thought*. London: Routledge.

Donlon, M., Ashman, O. and Levy, B. (2005). Creating a defence against television's ageism. *Journal of Social Issues*, 61, 307–19.

Dowd, J.J. (1980). Exchange rates and old people. *Journal of Gerontology*, 35(4), 596–602.

Durkheim, E. (1933). *The Division of Labor in Society* (G. Simpson trans.). New York: Free Press.

Dykstra, P.A. and Komter, A.E. (2006). Structural characteristics of Dutch kin networks. In P.A. Dykstra, A.E. Komter, T.C.M. Knijn, A.C. Liefbroer and C.H. Mulder (Eds), *Family Solidarity in the Netherlands* (pp. 21–421). Amsterdam: Dutch University Press.

Eagle (1994). 'A view from the eyrie'. Editorial. *Eagle*, 2, 6.

Eastman, M. (1984). *Old Age Abuse*. London: Age Concern.

Edmunds, J. and Turner, B. S. (Eds) (2002). *Generational Consciousness, Narrative and Politics*. Lanham, Boulder, New York and Oxford: Rowman and Littlefield.

Edmunds, J. and Turner, B. S. (2005). Global generations: Social change in the twentieth century. *The British Journal of Sociology*, 56(4), 559–77.

Elder G.H., Jr. (1974). *Children of the Great Depression*. Chicago: UCP.

Elder G.H., Jr. (1980). Adolescence in historical perspective. In J. Adelson (Ed.), *Handbook of Adolescent Psychology* (pp. 3–46). New York: Wiley.

Elder, G.H., Jr. (1985). Perspectives on the life course. In G. H., Jr. Elder (Ed.), *Life Course Dynamics: Trajectories and Transitions, 1968–1980* (pp. 23–49). Ithaca, NY: Cornell University Press.

Elder, G.H., Jr. (1994). Time, human agency, and social change: Perspectives on the life course. *Social Psychology Quarterly*, 57(1), 4–15.

Elder, G. H., Jr. and Caspi, A. (1990). Studying the lives in a changing society: Sociological and personological explorations. In A.I. Rabin, R.A. Zucker and S. Frank (Eds), *Studying Persons and Lives* (pp. 201–47). New York: Springer.

Elliot, A. (2002). *Psychoanalytic Theory*. Basingstoke: Palgrave.

Erikson, E.H. (1959). *Identity and the Life Cycle*. New York: International University Press.

Esping-Andersen, G. (1990). *The Three Worlds of Welfare Capitalism*. Princeton, NJ: Princeton University Press.

Esping-Andersen, G. (1999). *Social Foundations of Postindustrial Economies*. New York: Oxford University Press.

Estes, C.L. (1979). *The Aging Enterprise*. San Francisco: Jossey-Bass.

Estes, C.L. (1993). The aging enterprise revisited. *The Gerontologist*, 33(3), 292–98.

Estes, C.L., Linkins, K. and Binney, E. (2001). *Critical Perspective on Aging: The Political and Moral Economy of Growing Old*. Nove York: Baywood Publishing Company, pp. 117–34.

Estes, C.L. and Mahakian, J. (2001). The political economy of productive aging. In N. Morrow-Howell, J. Hinterlong and M.W. Sherraden (Eds), *Productive Aging: Concepts and Challenges* (pp. 197–213). Baltimore: Maryland, The Johns Hopkins University Press.

Estes, C.L., Biggs, S. and Phillipson, C. (2003). *Social Theory, Social Policy, and Ageing: A Critical Introduction*. Berkshire: Open University Press.

Eurobarometer (2008). *Health and Long Term Care in the European Union*. http://ec.europa. eu/public_opinion/archives/ebs/ebs_283_en.pdf.

European Commission (2005). *Confronting Demographic Change: A New Solidarity Between the Generations*. Green Paper, Commission of the European Communities. http://ec.europa.eu/employment_social/news/2005/mar/comm2005–94_en.pdf (Retrieved 17/8/08).

European Commission (2008). *Protecting the Dignity of Dependent Older People*. Comm. Memo. 17 March 2008. p. 5.

EUROSTAT (2007). *Living Conditions in Europe – Data 2002–2005*. Luxembourg: Office for Official Publications of the European Communities.

Evandrou, M. and Glaser, K. (2004). Family, work and quality of life: Changing economic and social roles through the lifecourse. *Ageing and Society*, 24(5), 771–91.

Evans, S. and Garner, J. (2004). *Talking Over the Years: A Handbook of Dynamic Psychotherapy with Older Adults*. London: Brunner-Routledge.

Faimberg, H. (2005). *The Telescoping of Generations: Listening to the Narcissistic Links Between Generations*. London: Routledge.

Featherstone, M. and Hepworth, M. (1989). Ageing and old age: Reflections on the post-modern life course. In B. Bytheway (Ed.), *Becoming and Being Old: Sociological Approaches to Later Life* (pp. 143–57). London: Sage.

Featherstone, M. and Hepworth, M. (1991). The mask of ageing and the postmodern lifecourse. In M. Featherstone, M. Hepworth and B. Turner (Eds), *The Body, Social Processes and Cultural Theory* (pp. 371–89). London: Sage.

Finch, J. (1995). Responsibilities, obligations and commitments. In I. Allen and E. Perkins (Eds), *The Future of Family Care for Older People* (pp. 51–64). London: HMSO.

Finch, J. and Mason, J. (1993). *Negotiating family responsibilities*. London: Tavistock/Routledge.

Fine, D.M. (2007). *A Caring Society? Care and the Dilemmas of Human Service in the 21st Century*. New York: MacMillan.

Fingerman, K.L. (2001). The paradox of a distant closeness: Intimacy in parent/child ties. *Generations*, 25(2), 26–33.

Fingerman, K.L., Hay, E.L. and Birditt, K.S. (2004). The best of ties, the worst of ties: Close problematic and ambivalent social relationships. *Journal of Marriage and Family*, 66(3), 792–808.

Fingerman, K.L., Chen, P. C., Hay, E.L., Cichy K.E. and Lefkovitz, E.S. (2006). Ambivalent reactions in the parent and offspring relationship. *The Journal of Gerontology*, Series B, 61(3), 152–60.

Fisher, B.J. (1992). Successful aging and life satisfaction: A pilot study for conceptual clarification. *Journal of Aging Studies*, 6, 191–202.

Fisher, P.P. (1995). *More Than Movement for Fit to Frail Older Adults: Creative Activities for the Body, Mind, and Spirit*. Baltimore: Health Professions Press.

Foucault, M. (1976/1981). *Discipline and Punish.* London: Penguin.

Foucault, M. (1977). *The History of Sexuality.* Vol 1. London: Penguin.

Frankenberger, K. (2002). Adolescent egocentrism: A comparison among adolescents and adults. *Journal of Adolescence*, 23(3), 343–54.

Freedman, M. (1999). *The Kindness of Strangers: Adult Mentors, Urban Youth, and the New Voluntarism.* New York: Cambridge University Press.

Freud, S. (1909/1962). *Two Short Accounts of Psychoanalysis*. London: Penguin.

Freud, S. (1936). *Civilization and its Discontents.* New York: Norton.

Fried, L.P., Freedman, M., Endres, T., Rebok, G.W., Carlson, M.C., Seeman, T.E., Tielsch, J., Glass, T.A., Wasik, B., Frick, K.D., Ialongo, N. and Zeger, S. (2002). *The Experience Corps: A Social Model for Health Promotion, Generativity, and Decreasing Structural Lag for Older Adults.* Symposium Presented at the 53rd Annual Meeting of the Gerontological Society of America. November 17–21, Washington, DC.

Friedberg, L. (2007). *The Recent Trend Toward Later Retirement.* CRR Issue in Brief No. 9. Chestnut Hill, MA: Center for Retirement Research at Boston College.

Fries, J.F. (1990). Medical perspectives upon successful aging. In P.B. Baltes and M.M. Baltes (Eds), *Successful Aging: Perspectives from the Behavioral Sciences* (pp. 35–49). New York: Cambridge University Press.

Fries, J.F. (2002). Successful aging – an emerging paradigm of gerontology. *Clinics in Geriatric Medicine*, 18, 371–82.

Frosh, S. (2003). Psychosocial studies and psychology: Is a critical approach emerging? *Human Relations*, 56(12), 1545–67.

Frost, S. and Hoggett, P. (2008). Human agency and social suffering. *Critical Social Policy*, 28(4), 438–60.

Gaalen, R., Dykstra, P. and Komter, A. (2010). Where is the exit? Intergenerational ambivalence and relationship quality in high contact ties. *Journal of Aging Studies*, 24(2), 105–14.

Gauthier, M. (2008). Insertion Professionnelle des Policiers des Générations X et Y. *Bilan Raisonné de la Littérature*, Document produit à la demande de l'Ecole nationale de police du Québec, Observatoire jeunes et société, Québec, 2008.

Generations United (2002). *Young and Old Serving Together: Meeting Community Needs through Intergenerational Partnerships.* www.epa.gov/aging/listening /2003/pdf/balt_ dbutt (Retrieved 9/3/09).

Generations United (2006). *Intergenerational Shared Sites: Making the Case.* www.gu.org/ documents/A0/GU-GeneralFactSheetJune.pdf

Generations United (undated). *Defining Intergenerational Programming.* Consulted on October 1, 2007 at http://www.gu.org/IG_Ov8191324.asp.

Gerstel, N. and Gallagher, S.K. (2001). Men's caregiving – Gender and the contingent character of care. *Gender and Society*, 15(2), 197–217.

Giancola, F. (2006). The generation gap: More myth than reality. *Human Resources Planning*, 29(4), 32–37.

Giarruso, R., Silverstein, M., Gans, D. and Bengtson, V.L. (2005). Ageing parents and ageing children: New perspectives on intergenerational relationships. In M.L. Johnson (Ed.), *The Cambridge Handbook of Age and Ageing* (pp. 413–21). Cambridge: Cambridge University Press.

Gibson, D. (1996). Broken down by age and gender: 'The problem of old women' redefined. *Gender and Society*, 10(4), 433–48.

Gigliotti, C.M., Morris, M., Smock, S., Jarrott, S.E. and Graham, B. (2005). Supporting community through an intergenerational summer program involving persons with dementia and pre-school children. *Educational Gerontology*, 31, 425–41.

Gilleard, C. (2004). Cohorts and generations in the study of social change. *Social Theory and Health*, 2, 106–109.

Gilleard, C. (2008). A murderous ageism? Age, death and Dr. Shipman. *Journal of Aging Studies*, 22(1), 88–95.

Gilleard, C. and Higgs, P. (2000). *Cultures of Ageing: Self, Citizen and the Body.* Malaysia: Pearson Education.

Gilleard, C. and Higgs, P. (2005). *Contexts of Ageing: Class, Cohort and Community.* Cambridge: Polity Press.

Gingold, R. (1999). *Successful Aging.* Melbourne: Oxford University Press.

Glass, T.A. (2003). Assessing the success of successful aging. *Annals of Internal Medicine*, 139(5), 1, 382–83.

Glendenning, F. (1993). What is elder abuse and neglect. In P. Decalmer and F. Glendenning, (Eds.), *The Mistreatment of Elderly People* (pp. 1–34). London: Sage.

Glenn, E.N. (2000). Creating a caring society. *Contemporary Sociology*, 29(1), 84–94.

Goff, K. (2004). Senior to senior: living lessons. *Educational Gerontology*, 30, 205–17.

Georgen, T. (2007). Abuse and neglect of elderly people in residential care. *Research in Legal Medicine*, 27, 367–92.

Graham, H. (1983). Caring: A labour of love. In J. Finch and G. Dulcie (Eds), *A Labour of Love: Women, Work and Caring* (pp. 13–30). London: Routledge.

Granville, G. and Hatton-Yeo, A. (2002). Intergenerational engagement in the UK: A framework for creating inclusive communities. In M. Kaplan, N. Henkin and A. Kusano (Eds), *Linking Lifetimes: A Global View of Intergenerational Exchange* (pp. 193–208). Lanham, MD: University Press of America.

Grenier, A. (2007). Crossing age and generational boundaries: Exploring intergenerational research encounters. *Journal of Social Issues*, 63(4), 713–27.

Gruber, J. and Wise, D.A. (2001). *An International Perspective on Policies for an Aging Society.* NBER Wokring Paper No. 8103. Cambridge, MA: National Bureau of Economic Research.

Grundy, E. and Henretta, J.C. (2006). Between elderly parents and adult children: A new look at the intergenerational care provided by the 'sandwich generation'. *Ageing and Society*, 26(5), 707–22.

Gubrium, J. and Wallace, J. (1990). Who theorises age? *Ageing and Society*, 10(2), 131–49.

Hagestad, G.O. (2003). Interdependent lives and relationships in changing times: A life course view of families and aging. In R. Settersten (Ed.), *Invitation to the Life Course Toward New Understanding of Later Life* (pp. 135–59). Amityville, NY: Baywood.

Hagestad, G.O. and Uhlenberg, P. (2005). The social separation of old and young: A root of ageism. *Journal of Social Issues*, 61(2), 343–60.

Hagestad, G.O. and Uhlenberg, P. (2006). Should we be concerned about age segregation? Some theoretical and empirical explorations. *Research on Aging*, 28(6), 638–53.

Hagestad, G.O. and Uhlenberg, P. (2007). The impact of demographic changes on relations between age groups and generations: A comparative perspective. In K. W. Schaie and P.

Uhlenberg (Eds), *Social structures: Demographic Change and the Well-Being of Older Adults* (pp. 239–61). New York, NY: Springer.

Halperin, D. (2007). *Stress Feelings Related to Role Strain and Role Conflict and their Impact on Marital Quality of Working Women Caring for an Elderly Parent.* MA thesis, Haifa, Israel: University of Haifa (Hebrew, English abstract).

Hanks, R.S. and Icenogle, M. (2001). Preparing for an age-diverse workforce: Intergenerational service-learning in social gerontology and business curricula. *Educational Gerontology*, 27(1), 49–70.

Hanks, R.S. and Pomzetti, J.J. (2004). Family studies and intergenerational studies: Intersections and opportunities. *Journal of Intergenerational Relationships*, 2(3/4), 5–22.

Hareven, T.K. (1994). Aging and generational relations: A historical and life course perspective. *Annual Review of Sociology*, 20, 437–61.

Hareven, T.K. (1996). Introduction: Aging and generational relations over the life course. In T.K. Hareven (Ed.), *Aging and Generational Relations Life-Course and Cross Cultural Perspectives.* New York: Aldine De Gruyter.

Harper, S. (2005). Grandparenthood. In M.L. Johnson (Ed.), *The Cambridge Handbook of Age and Ageing.* (pp. 422–28). Cambridge: Cambridge University Press.

Harreveld, F., Rutjens, B., Rotteveel, M., Nordgren, L. and van Der Pligt, J. (2009). Ambivalence and decisional conflict as a cause of psychological discomfort: Feeling tense before jumping off the fence. *Journal of Experimental Social Psychology*, 45(1), 167–73.

Hatton-Yeo, A. (Ed.) (2006). *Intergenerational Programmes: An Introduction and Examples of Practice.* Stoke-on-Trent: The Beth Johnson Foundation.

Hatton-Yeo, A. and Ohsako, T. (Eds) (2001). *Intergenerational Programmes: Public Policy and Research Implications and International Perspectives* (pp. 9–17). Hamburg, Germany: UNESCO Institute for Education.

Hayes, C. (2003). An observational study in developing an intergenerational shared site program: Challenges and insights. *Journal of Intergenerational Relationships*, 1(1), 113–32.

Hazan, H. (2011). Gerontological autism: Terms of accountability in the cultural study of the category of the fourth age. *Ageing and Society*, (61)1.

Help the Aged (2000). *'Our Future Health'* campaign literature. London: Help the Aged.

Hendricks, J. (2004). Public policy and old age identity. *Journal of Aging Studies*, 18(3), 245–60.

Hendricks, J. and Achenbaum, A. (1999). Historical developments of theories of aging. In V. L. Bengtson, and K.W. Schie (Eds), *Handbook of Theories of Aging* (pp. 21–39). NY: Springer.

Henkin, N. and Kengson, E. (Eds) (1998–1999). Keeping the promise: Intergenerational strategies for strengthening the social compact [Special issue]. *Generations, Journal of the American Society on Aging*, 22(4).

Henz, U. (2006). Informal caregiving at working age: Effects of job characteristics and family configuration. *Journal of Marriage and the Family*, 68(2), 411–29.

Hepworth, M. (2004). Embodied agency, decline and the mask of ageing. In E. Tulle (Ed.), *Old Age and Agency* (pp. 125–36). NY: Nova.

Hildon, Z., Smith, G., Netuveli, G. and Blane, D. (2008). Understanding adversity and resilience at older ages. *Sociology of Heath and Illness*. 30(5), 1–15.

Hinterlong, J., Morrow-Howell, N. and Sherraden, M. (2001). Productive aging: Principles and perspectives. In N. Morrow-Howell, J. Hinterlong and M. Sherraden (Eds), *Productive Aging: Concepts and Challenge.* Baltimore: Johns Hopkins.

Hoff, A. and Tesch-Roemer, C. (2007). Family relations and aging: Substantial changes since the middle of the last century. In H. W. Wahl, C. Tesch-Roemer and A. Hoff (Eds), *New Dynamics in Old Age: Individual, Environment and Societal Perspectives* (pp. 65–84). New York, NY: Baywood Publishing.

Holstein, J.A. and Gubrium, J.F. (2000). *The Self We Live By*. Oxford: Oxford University Press.

Horl, J. (2007). Social construction of violence in old age. *Journal of Adult Protection.* 9(1), 33–38.

Howe, N. and Strauss, W. (2007). The next 20 years: How customer and workforce attitudes will evolve. *Harvard Business Review* (July–August): 41–52.

HRSDC (2008). *Comparative Summary of National Prevalence Studies*. Ottawa: HRSDC.

Hudson, M.F. (1991). Elder mistreatment: A taxonomy with definitions by Delphi. *Journal of Elder Abuse and Neglect*, 3(2), 1–20.

Hughes, M.E. and O'Rand, A.M. (2004). *The Lives and Times of the Baby Boom*. Census 2000 Monograph. New York: Russell Sage Foundation/Washington DC: Population Reference Bureau.

Hummert, M., Garstka,T., Shaner, J. and Strahm, S. (1994). Stereotypes of the elderly held by young, middle aged and elderly adults. *Journal of Gerontology*, 49(5), 240–49.

Hussein, S., Manthorpe, J. and Penhale, B. (2007). Public perceptions of the neglect and mistreatment of older people: Findings of a UK survey. *Ageing and Society*, 27(6), 919–40.

Iborra, I. (2008). *Elder Abuse in the Family in Spain*. Doc 14. Valencia: Centro Reina Sofia.

Ickes, W. (1997). *Empathic Accuracy*. New York: The Guilford Press.

International Labour Office (ILO) (2000). Income security and social protection in a changing world. *World Labour Report*. Geneva: ILO.

Irwin, S. (1998). Age, generation and inequality. *British Journal of Sociology*, 49(2), 305–10.

Jackson, J.S., Brown, E., Antonucci, T. and Daatland, S.O. (2005). Ethnic diversity in aging, multi-cultural society. In M.L. Johnson, V.L. Bengtson, P.G. Coleman and T.B.L. Kirkwood (Eds), *The Cambridge Handbook of Age and Ageing* (pp. 476–81). Cambridge, England: Cambridge University Press.

Jackson, V. (1996). *The Abusive Elder*. Binghampton, NY: Haworth.

Jaques, E. (1965). Death and the midlife crisis. *International Journal of Psychoanalysis.* 46(94), 507–14.

Jarrott, S.E. (2007). *Tried and true: A guide to successful intergenerational activities at shared site programs*. Washington, DC: Generations United. [Electronic version available at www.gu.org].

Jarrott, S.E. and Bruno, K. (2003). Intergenerational activities involving persons with dementia: An observational assessment. *American Journal of Alzheimer's and Related Diseases*, 18(1), 31–38.

Jarrott, S.E. and Bruno, K. (2007). Shared site intergenerational programs: A case study. *Journal of Applied Gerontology*, 26(3), 239–57.

Jarrott, S.E., Gigliotti, C.M. and Smock, S.A. (2006). Where do we stand? Testing the foundation of a shared site intergenerational program. *Journal of Inter-Generational Relationships*, 4(2), 73–92.

Jarrott, S.E., Morris, M., Kemp, A.J. and Stremmel, A. (2004, November). *Intergenerational Cross-Training Partners: Collaboration at a Shared Site Community*. Paper presented at the meetings of the Gerontological Society of America, Washington, D.C

Johansson, B., Karlsson, C., Backman, M. and Juusola, P. (2007). *Paper No.106. The Lisbon Agenda From 2000 to 2010.* http://www.infra.kth.se/cesis/documents/WP106. pdf (Retrieved (16/5/10)

Johnson, T. (1986). Critical issues in the definition of elder mistreatment. In K.A. Pillemer and R.S. Wolf (Eds), *Elder Abuse: Conflict in the Family* (pp. 167–96). Dover Mass: Auburn House.

Juklestad, O. (2001). Institutional care for older people: The dark side. *Journal of Adult Protection*, 3(2), 32–41.

Juklestad, O. and Espas, A. (2006). Elder protection services in Norway. Paper presented to European Commission AGIS Network Conference 'Violence against and grave neglect of elders under institutional and care conditions'. Cologne: May 2006.

Jung, C.G. (1931/1967). *Collected Works.* Vol. 7. London: Routledge.

Jung, C.G. (1931). *The Aims of Psychotherapy.* London: Routledge.

Jung, C.G. (1932/1967). *Collected Works.* Vol. 9. London: Routledge.

Jung, C.G. (1939/1967). *Collected Works.* Vol 16. London: Routledge.

Jung, C. G. (1961). *Memories, Dreams, Reflections.* London: Routledge.

Jurkiewicz C.E. and Brown R.G. (1998). Gen X-ers vs. boomers vs matures: Generational comparisons of public employee motivation. *Review of Public Personnel Administration*, 18(4), 18–37.

Kalmijn, M. and Saraceno, C. (2008). A comparative perspective on intergenerational support. *European Societies*, 10(3), 479–508.

Kaplan, M. and Chadha, N. (2004). Intergenerational programs and practices: A conceptual framework and an Indian context. *Indian Journal of Gerontology*, 18(3–4).

Katz, R. and Lowenstein, A. (2010). Theoretical perspectives on intergenerational solidarity, conflict and ambivalence. In Misa Izuhara (Ed.), *Ageing and Intergenerational Relations* (pp. 29–57). The Policy Press, UK

Katz, R., Gur-Yaish, N. and Lowenstein, A. (2010). Motivation to provide help to older parents in Norway, Spain and Israel. *International Journal of Aging and Human Development*, 71(4), 283–303.

Katz, R., Lowenstein, A., Phillips, J. and Daatland, S.O. (2005). Theorizing intergenerational family relations. Solidarity, conflict and ambivalence in cross-national contexts. In V.L. Bengtson, A.C. Acock, K.R. Allen, P. Dilworth-Anderson and D. Klein (Eds), *Sourcebook of Family Theory and Research* (pp. 393–402). Thousand Oaks: Sage.

Katz, R., Daatland, S.O., Lowenstein, A., Bazo, M.T., Herlofson, K., Mehlausen-Hassoen, D., Prilutzky, D. and Ancizu, I. (2003). Family norms and preferences in intergenerational relations: A comparative perspective. In V. L. Bengtson and A. Lowenstein (Eds), *Global Aging and Challenges to Families* (pp. 305–26). New York and Berlin: Aldine De Gruyter.

Katz, S. (2000). Busy bodies: activity, aging and the management of everyday life. *Journal of Aging Studies*, 14(2), 135–52.

Kaufman, G. and Elder, G. (2002). Revisiting age identity. *Journal of Aging Studies*, 16(2), 169–76.

Kingston, P. and Penhale, B. (1995). *Family Violence and the Caring Professions.* London: Macmillan.

Kinsella, K. (2000). Demographic dimensions of global aging. *Journal of Family Issues*, 21(5), 541–58.

Knight, B. (1996). *Psychotherapy with Older Adults.* Newbury Park, CA: Sage.

Knight, T. and Ricciardelli, L.A. (2003). Successful aging: Perceptions of adults aged between 70 and 101 years. *The International Journal of Aging and Human Development*, 56(3), 223–46.

Kohli, M. (1986). The world we forgot: A historical review of the life course. In V.W. Marshall (Ed.), *Later Life: The Social Psychology of Aging*. London: Sage.

Kohli, M. (1996). *The Problem of Generations: Family, Economy, Politics*. Collegium Budapest, Public Lectures Series No. 14. Budapest: Collegium Budapest.

Kohli, M. (2005). Generational changes and generational equity. In M.L. Johnson (Ed.), *The Cambridge Handbook of Age and Ageing* (pp. 518–26). Cambridge: Cambridge University Press.

Kohli, M. (2007). The institutionalization of the life course: Looking back to look ahead. *Research in Human Development*, 4(3–4), 253–71.

Kuehne, V.S. (1992). Older adults in intergenerational programs: What are their experiences really like? *Activities, Adaptation and Aging*, 16(4), 49–67.

Kuehne, V.S. (Ed.), (2003). The state of our art: Intergenerational program research and evaluation. Part one. *Journal of Intergenerational Relationships*, 1(1), 145–61.

Kunemund, H. and Rein, M. (1999). There is more to receiving than needing: Theoretical arguments and empirical explorations of crowding-in and crowding-out. *Ageing and Society*, 19, 93–121.

Kupperschmidt, B.R. (2000). Multigeneration employees: Strategies for effective management. *Health Care Manager*, 19(1), 65–76.

Lamura, G., Mnich, E., Nolan, M., Wojszel, B., Krevers, B., Mestheneos, L. and Dohner, H. (2008). Family carers' experiences using support services in Europe: Empirical evidence from the EUROFAMCARE study. *The Gerontologist*, 48(6), 752–71.

Larkin, E. (1998–1999). The intergenerational response to childcare and after-school care. *Generations*, 22(4), 33–36.

Larkin, P. (1971). *Collected Works*. London: Faber and Faber.

Laws, G. (1997). Embodiment and emplacement. *International Journal of Aging and Human Development*, 40(4), 253–80.

Leitner, S. (2003). Varieties of familialims: The caring function of the family in comparative perspective. *European Societies*, 19, 93–121.

Levi, B.R. and Banaji, M.R. (2002). Implicit ageism. In T.D. Nelson (Ed.), *Ageism: Stereotyping and Prejudice Against Older Persons* (pp. 49–76). Cambridge, Mass: MIT Press.

Levkoff, S.E., Chee, Y.K. and Noguchi, S. (2001). *Aging in Good Health: Multidisciplinary Perspectives*. New York: Springer.

Lieberman, M.A. and Fisher, L. (1999). The effects of family conflict resolution and decision making on the provision of help for an elder with Alzheimer's disease. *Gerontologist*, 39(2), 159–66.

Litwak, E. (1985). *Helping the Elderly: The Complementary Roles of Informal Networks and Formal Systems*. New York: Guilford Press.

Logan, J. and Spitze, G. (1996). *Family Ties: Enduring Relations Between Parents and Their Grown Children*. Philadelphia: Temple University Press.

Lorenz-Meyer, D. (2001). The politics of ambivalence. *Gender Institute New Working Paper Series 2* (pp. 1–24).

Lowenstein, A. (2003). Contemporary later-life family transitions: Revisiting theoretical perspectives on aging and the family – toward a family identity framework. In S. Biggs, A. Lowenstein and J. Hendricks (Eds), *The Need for Theory: Critical Approaches to Social Gerontology* (pp. 105–26). Amityville, New York: Baywood Publishing Co., Inc.

Lowenstein, A. (2005). Global aging and the challenges to families. In M. Johnson, V.L. Bengtson, P.G. Coleman and T. Kirkwood (Eds), *Cambridge Handbook on Age and Aging* (pp. 403–13). Cambridge: Cambridge University Press.

Lowenstein, A. (2007). Solidarity-conflict and ambivalence: Testing two conceptual frameworks and their impact on quality of life for older family members. *Journal of Gerontology: Social Sciences*, 62B: S100–S7.

Lowenstein, A. and Daatland, S.O. (2006). Filial norms and family support to the old-old (75+) in a comparative cross-national context (the OASIS study). *Ageing & Society*, 26(5), 723–43.

Lowenstein, A. and Doron, I. (2008). Times of transition: Elder abuse and neglect in Israel. *Journal of Elder Abuse and Neglect*, 20(2), 181–206

Lowenstein, A. and Katz, R. (2000). Coping with caregiving in the rural Arab family in Israel. *Marriage and Family Review*, 30(1), 179–97.

Lowenstein, A. and Katz, R. (2010). Family and age in global perspectives. In Chris Phillipson and Dale Dannefer (Eds), *Handbook of Social Gerontology* (pp. 190–201). London: Sage Publications.

Lowenstein, A., Katz, R. and Daatland, S.O. (2004). Filial norms and intergenerational support in a comparative cross-national perspective. *Annual Review of Gerontology and Geriatrics*, 24, 200–24.

Lowenstein, A., Katz, R. and Gur-Yaish, N. (2007). Reciprocity in parent child exchange and life satisfaction among the elderly: A cross national perspective. *Journal of Social Issues*, 63(4), 865–84.

Lowenstein, A., Katz, R. and Gur-Yaish, N. (2008). Cross national variations in elder care: Antecedents and outcomes. In M. E. Szinovacz and A. Davey (Eds), *Caregiving Contexts* (pp. 93–114). New York: Spring Publishing Co.

Lowenstein, A., Eisikovits, Z., Band-Winterstein, T. and Enosh, G. (2009). Is elder abuse and neglect a social phenomenon? Data from the First National Prevalence Survey in Israel. *Journal of Elder Abuse and Neglect*, 21(3), 253–60.

Luescher, K. (1998). Forcierte Ambivalenzen: Ehescheidung als Herausforderung an die *Generationenbeziehungen unter Erwachsenen*. Working paper 29. University of Konstnaz: Germany.

Luescher, K. (2002). Intergenerational ambivalence: Further steps in theory and research. *Journal of Marriage and Family*, 64(3), 585–93.

Luescher, K. and Pillemer, K. (1998). Intergenerational ambivalence: A new approach to the study of parent-child relations in later life. *Journal of Marriage and the Family*, 60(2), 413–25.

Lynnott, R.L. and Lynnott, P.P. (1996). Tracing the course of theoretical development in the sociology of ageing. *The Gerontologist*, 36(6), 749–60.

McAdams, D. (1985). *Power, Intimacy and the Lifestory*. Homewood, IL: Dorsey.

McAdams, D. (1993). *The Stories We Live By*. New York: Morrow.

McAdams, D. (1997). The case for unity in the post modern self. In R. Ashmore and L. Jussim (Eds), *Self and Identity*. Oxford: OUP.

McAdams, D. (2001). Generativity in midlife. In M. Lachman (Ed.), *Handbook of Midlife Development* (pp. 395–447). New York: Wiley.

McAdams, D. and De St. Aubin, E. (Eds) (1998). *Generativity and Adult Development: How and Why We Care for the Next Generation*. Washington, DC: American Psychological Association.

McCluskey, U. and Hooper, C.A. (2000) *Psychodynamic Perspectives on Abuse*. London: Jessica Kingsley.

McCreadie, C. and Biggs, S. (2006). Elder abuse: The last taboo? *Geriatric Medicine*, 36(6), 21–25.

McDaniel, S.A. (2008). The 'Growing Legs' of Generation and a Policy Construct: Reviving its *Family Meaning*. Paper presented for: Aging, families and households in global perspective, Boston, May 19–23, 2008.

McDonald, L., Donahue, P. and Moore, B. (1998). *The Economic Casualties of Retiring to Caregive* (No. 28). Hamilton, ON: Independence and Economic Security of the Older Population.

McDonald, L., Donahue, P. and Moore, B. (forthcoming). The economic hardships after care is over. *Journal of Gerontology: Social Sciences*.

McMullin, J.A., Comeau, T.D. and Jovic, E. (2007). Generational affinities and discourses of difference: A case study of highly skilled information technology workers. *The British Journal of Sociology*, 58(2), 297–316.

Maccallum, J., Palmer, D., Wright, P., Cumming Potvin, W., Northcote, J., Booker, M. and Tero, C. (2006). *Community Building Through Intergenerational Exchange Programs*. Australia: National Youth Affairs Research Scheme.

Mancini, J.A. and Blieszner, R. (1989). Aging parents and adult children: Research themes in intergenerational relations. *Journal of Marriage and the Family*, 51(2), 275–90.

Manheimer, R.J. (1997). Generations learning together. In K. Brabazon and R. Disch (Eds), *Intergenerational Approaches in Aging*, pp. 79–91. New York: The Haworth Press.

Mannheim, K. (1928/1952). The problem of generations. In P. Kecskemeti (Ed.), *Essays on the Sociology of Knowledge* (pp. 276–319). London: Routledge and Kegal Paul.

Mannheim, K. (1952). *Essays on the Sociology of Knowledge*. New York: John Villey.

Mannheim, K. (1998). *Saggi di Sociologia Della Cultura*. Armando Editore.

Marcoen, A., Coleman, P. and O'Hanlon, A. (2007). Psychological ageing. In J. Bond, S. Peace, F. Dittmann-Kohli and G. Westerhoff (Eds), *Ageing in Society* (pp. 38–67). London: Sage.

Marcuse, H. (1964). *One Dimensional Man*. London: Abacus.

Marshall, V.W. (2007). Advancing the sociology of ageism. *Social Forces*, 86(1), 257.

Marshall, V.W. (forthcoming). Global aging and families: Some policy concerns about the global aging perspective. In M. Silverstein (Ed.), *From Generation to Generation: Continuity and Discontinuity in Aging Families*. Baltimore: The Johns Hopkins University Press.

Marshall, V.W. and Marshall, J.G. (1999). Age and changes in work: Causes and contrasts. *Ageing International*, 25(2), 46–68.

Marshall, V.W. and Taylor, P. (2005). Restructuring the life course: Work and retirement. In M.L. Johnson, V.L. Bengtson, P.G. Coleman and T.B.L. Kirkwood (Eds), *The Cambridge Handbook of Age and Ageing* (pp. 572–82). Cambridge: Cambridge University Press.

Marshall, V.W. and Wells, A.L. (forthcoming). Generational relations and the workplace: A critique of the concept. In P. Taylor (Ed.), *Older Workers in an Ageing Society: Critical Topics in Research and Policy*. Camberly: Edward Elgar.

Marshall, V.W., Matthews, S.H. and Rosenthal, C.J. (1993). Elusiveness of family life. *Annual Review of Gerontology and Geriatrics*, 13, 39–72.

Marshall, V.W., Rosenthal, C. and Dacink, J. (1987). Older parents expectations for filial support. *Social Justice Research*, 1(4), 405–24.

Marshall, V.W., Heinz, W.R., Kruger, H. and Verma, A. (Eds) (2001). *Restructuring Work and the Life Course*. Toronto: University of Toronto Press.

Martens, A., Goldenberg, J.A. and Greenberg, J. (2005). A terror management perspective on ageism. *Journal of Social Issues*, 61(2), 223–39.

Martin, C.A. and Tulgan, B. (2001). *Managing Generation Y.* Amharst, MA: HRD Press.

Martin, C.A. and Tulgan, B. (2002). *Managing the Generation Mix.* Amherst, MA: HRD Press.

Marx, M.S., Pannell, A.R., Parpura-Gill, A. and Cohen-Mansfield, J. (2004). Direct observations of children at risk for academic failure: Benefits of an intergenerational visiting program. *Educational Gerontology*, 30, 663–75.

Mercken, C. (2003). Neighborhood-reminiscence: Integrating generations and cultures in the Netherlands. *Journal of Intergenerational Relationships: Programs, Policy, and Research.* 1(1): 81–94.

Merrill, D.M. (1996). Conflict and cooperation among adult siblings during the transition to the role of filial caregiver. *Journal of Social and Personal Relationships*, 13(3), 399–413.

Merz, E.M., Schuengel, C. and Schule, H.J. (2007). Intergenerational solidarity: An attachment perspective. *Journal of Aging Studies*, 21(1), 175–86.

Meshel, D.S. and McGlynn, R.P. (2004). Intergenerational contact, attitudes, and stereotypes of adolescents and older people. *Educational Gerontology*, 30, 457–79.

Middelcoop, P. (1985). *The Wise Old Man.* New York: Shambhala.

Millward, C. (1999). Caring for elderly parents. *Family Matters*, 52, 26–30.

Minkler, M. and Estes, C. (1998). *Critical Gerontology: Perspectives from Political and Moral Economy.* Amityville, New York: Baywood Publishing Company, Inc.

Minkler, M. and Robertson, A. (1991). The ideology of age-race wars. *Ageing and Society*, 11(1), 1–22.

Moody, H.R. (2001). Productive aging and the ideology of old age. In N. Morrow-Howell, J. Hinterlong and M. Sherraden (Eds), *Productive Aging: Concepts and Challenges.* Baltimore: Johns Hopkins.

Moody, H.R. (2008). Aging America and the boomer wars. *The Gerontologist*, 48(6), 839–44.

Morgan, J.N. (1986). Unpaid productive activity over the life course. In *America's Aging – Productive Roles in an Older Society* (pp. 73–109). Washington DC: Institute of Medicine/National Research Council.

Morgan, L. and Knukel, S. (1998). *Aging: The Social Context.* Thousand Oaks, CA: Pine Forge Press.

Morrison, B. and Ahmed, E. (Eds) (2006). Restorative justice and civil society. *Journal of Social Issues*, 62(2), 209–11.

Morrow-Howell, N., Hinterlong, J. and Sherraden, M. (2001). *Productive Aging: Concepts and Challenges.* Baltimore, MA: Johns Hopkins.

Mosher-Ashley, P. and Ball, P. (1999). Attitudes of college students toward elderly persons and their perceptions of themselves at age 75. *Educational Gerontology*, 25, 89–103.

Musil, C.M., Morris, D.L., Warner, C.B. and Saeid, H. (2003). Issues in caregivers' stress and providers' support. *Research on Aging*, 25(5), 505–26.

National Alliance for Caregivers/AARP. (2004). *Caregiving in the US.* Bethesda, MD.

National Center for Elder Abuse (2009). Washington DC: National Center on Elder Abuse. http://www.ncea.aoa.gov/ncearoot/Main_Site/index.aspx. Retrieved (15/6/10).

National Research Council (2003). *Elder Mistreatment: Abuse, Neglect and Exploitation in an Aging Society.*

National Service Framework for Older People. (2001). London: Department of Health.

National Service Framework for Older People Reviewed. (2005). London: Department of Health.

Neal, M.B. and Hammer, L.B. (2007). *Working Couples Caring for Children and Aging Parents.* Mahwah, NJ: Lawrence Erlbaum Associates.

Neugarten, B., Havighurst, R. and Tobin, S. (1968). Personality and patterns of aging. In B. Neugarten (Ed.), *Middle Age and Aging* (pp. 173–77). Chicago: University of Chicago Press.

Newman, S. (1997). History and evolution of intergenerational programs. In S. Newman, R. Ward, T. Smith, J. Wilson and J. McCrea. *Intergenerational Programs: Past, Present and Future* (pp. 55–79). Washington, DC: Taylor & Francis.

Newman, S. and Larimer, B. (1995). *Senior Citizen School Volunteer Program: Report on Cumulative Data 1988–1995.* Pittsburgh, PA: Generations Together, University of Pittsburgh.

Newman, S., Faux, R. and Larimer, B. (1997). Children's views of aging: Their attitudes and values. *The Gerontologist,* 37(3), 412–17.

Newman, S., Morris, G.A. and Streetman, H. (1999). Elder-child interaction analysis: An observation instrument for classrooms involving older adults as mentors, tutors or resource persons. In V.S. Kuehne (Ed.), *Intergenerational Programs: Understanding What We Have Created* (pp. 129–45). Binghamton: The Haworth Press.

Newman, S., Ward, C. and Smith, T. (1997). *Intergenerational Programs: Past, Present, and Future.* Washington, DC: Taylor & Francis.

Nicole-Drancourt, C. and Roulleau-Berger, L. (2001). *Les Jeunes et le Travail.* 1950–2000, Paris, Puf.

Nikander, P. (2009). Doing change and continuity: Age identity and the micro-macro divide. *Ageing and Society,* 29(6), 863–82.

Norrick, N. (2009). The construction of multiple identities in elderly narrator's stories. *Ageing and Society,* 29(6), 903–28.

Nye, F.I. and Rushing, W. (1969). Towards family measurement research. In J. Hadden and E. Borgatta (Eds), *Marriage and Family.* Illinois City: Peacock.

O'Hanlon, A. and Coleman, P. (2004). *Ageing and Development: Theories and Research.* London: Arnold.

O'Keeffe, M., Hills, A., Doyle, M., McCreadie, C., Scholes, S., Constantine, R., Tinker, A., Manthorpe, J., Biggs, S. and Erens, B. (2007). *UK Study of Abuse and Neglect of Older People: Prevalence Survey Report.* London: NatCen.

Ohsako, T. (2002). German pupils and Jewish seniors: Intergenerational dialogue as a framework for healing history. In M. Kaplan, N. Henkin and A. Kusano (Eds), *Linking Lifetimes: A Global View of Intergenerational Exchange* (pp. 209–19). Lanham, MD: University Press of America.

Olazabal, I. (2005). Interview with Francois Ricard: the Lyric generation. *Vital Aging,* 11(2), 3.

Olshansky, J., Carnes, B. and Butler, R. (2007). *Securing the Longevity Dividend.* Chicago, IL: Institute for Ethics and Emerging Technologies, July 23.

Organization for Economic Co-operation and Development (2006). *OECD Economic Surveys.* Paris: OECD.

Osborne, S.S. and Bullock, J.R. (2000). Intergenerational programming in action: Befrienders. *Educational Gerontology,* 26(2), 169–82.

Padilla, E. (2002). Intergenerational equity and sustainability. *Ecological Economy,* 41(1), 69–83.

Palmore, E.B. (1979). Predictors of successful aging. *The Gerontologist*, 19, 427–31.

Palmore, E.B. (1995). Successful aging. In G.L. Maddox (Ed.), *The Encyclopaedia of Aging*. New York: Springer.

Palmore, E.B. (1999). *Ageism: Negative and Positive*. New York: Springer.

Papalia, D.E. and Wendkos, O. (2006). *Human Development*. New York: McGraw Hill.

Papalia, D.E. and Olds, S.W. (2000). *Desenvolvimento Humano*, 7, ed. Porto Alegre: Artes Médicas.

Parrott, T.M. and Bengtson, V.L. (1999). The effects of earlier intergenerational affection, normative expectations, and family conflict on contemporary exchange of help and support. *Research on Aging*, 21(1), 73–105.

Paugam, S. (2000). *Le Salarié de la Précarité*, Paris: Puf.

Pavalko, E.K. and Henderson, K.A. (2006). Combining care work and paid work. *Research on Aging*, 28(3), 359–74.

Penning, M.J. (2002). Hydra revisited: Substituting formal for self and informal in-home care among older adults with disabilities. *Gerontologist*, 42(1), 4–16.

Penrod, J., Gueldner, S.H. and Poon, L.W. (2003). Managing multiple chronic health conditions in everyday life. In L.W. Poon, S.H. Gueldner and B.M. Sprouse (Eds), *Successful Aging and Adaptation With Chronic Diseases* (pp. 181–208). New York: Springer Publication.

Pezzin, E L., Pollak, A.R. and Schone, S.B. (2005). *Bargaining Power and Intergenerational Coresidence: Adult Children and their Disabled Elderly Parents*. Working paper Rockville.

Phelan, E.A., Anderson, L.A., Lacroix, A.Z. and Larson, E.B. (2004). Older adults' views of 'Successful Aging' – How do they compare with researchers' definitions? *American Geriatrics Society*, 52(2), 211–16.

Phillips, J., Ajrouch, K. and Hillcoat, S. (2010). *Key Concepts in Social Gerontology*. London: Sage.

Phillipson, C. (1998). *Reconstructing Ageing*. London: Sage.

Phillipson, C. (2003). From family groups to personal communities: Social capital and social change in the family life of older people. In V.L. Bengtson and A. Lowenstein (Eds), *Global Aging and Challenges to Families* (pp. 54–74). New York: Aldine De Gruyter.

Phillipson, C. (2010). Globalization, global ageing and intergenerational change. In M. Izuhara (Ed.), *Ageing and Intergenerational Relations: Family Reciprocity from a Global Perspective* (pp. 13–28). University of Bristol, UK: The Policy Press.

Phillipson, C. and Biggs, S. (2001). Population ageing: Critical Gerontology and the sociological tradition. *Education and Ageing*, 14(2), 165–76.

Phillipson, C., Leach, R., Money, A. and Biggs, S. (2008). Social and cultural constructions of ageing: The case of the baby boomers. *Sociological Research Online*, 13(3), 23–34.

Piaget, J. (1952). *The Origins of Intelligence in Children*. New York: International University Press.

Piercy, K.W. (1998). Theorizing about family caregiving: The role of responsibility. *Journal of Marriage and the Family*, 60(1), 109–18.

Pilcher, J. (1994). Mannheim's sociology of generations: An undervalued legacy. *The British Journal of Sociology*, 45(3), 481–95.

Pillemer, K.A. and Finkelhor, D. (1988). The prevalence of elder abuse: A random sample survey. *The Gerontologist*, 28(1), 51–57.

Pillemer, K.A. and Luescher, K. (Eds) (2004). *Intergenerational Ambivalences: New Perspectives on Parent-Child Relations in Later Life* (pp. 23–62). Oxford: Elsevier.

Pillemer, K.A. and Moore, D. (1989). Abuse of patients in nursing homes: Findings from a survey of staff. *The Gerontologist*, 29(3), 314–20.

Pillemer K.A. and Suitor, J.J. (1991). Will I even escape my child's problems? Effects of adult children's problems on elderly parents. *Journal of Marriage and the Family*, 53(3), 585–94.

Pillemer, K.A. and Suitor, J.J. (2002). Explaining mothers' ambivalence toward their adult children. *Journal of Marriage and the Family*, 64(3), 602–13.

Pillemer, K.A. and Wolf, R.S. (Eds) (1986). *Elder Abuse: Conflict in the Family*. Dover Mass: Auburn House.

Pillemer, K.A., Suitor, J., Mock, S., Sabir, M., Prado, T. and Sechrist, J. (2007). Capturing the complexity of intergenerational relations: Exploring ambivalence within later-life families. *Journal of Social Issues*, 63(4), 793–808.

Pincus, L. and Dare, C. (1978). *Secrets in the Family*. London: Faber.

Piotet, F. (2007). *Emploi et Travail. Le Grand Écart*. Paris. Armand Colin.

Podnieks, E. (2007). *Worldview Environmental Scan*. http://www.inpea.net/reportsresources/reports.html (Retrieved 8/3/10).

Powell, J. and Biggs, S. (2003). Foucaultian Gerontology: A methodology for understanding ageing. *Electronic Journal of Sociology*, 7(2), 1–9.

Power, M. and Maluccio, A. (1998–1999). Intergenerational approaches to helping families at risk. *Generations*, 22(4), 37–42.

Pruchno, R.A., Burant, C.J. and Peters, N.D. (1997). Typologies of care-giving families: Family congruence and individual well-being. *The Gerontologist*, 32(2), 157–67.

Qureshi, H. and Walker, A. (1989). *The Caring Relationships: Elderly People and their Families*. Basingstoke: MacMillan.

Riffault, H. and Tchernia, J.F. (2002). Les Européens et le travail: un rapport plus personnel. *Futuribles*, 227, 63–77.

Roberts, R.E.L. and Bengtson, V.L. (1990). Is intergenerational solidarity a unidimensional construct? A second test of a formal model. *Journal of Gerontology: Social Sciences*, 45, S12–S20.

Roberts, R.E.L., Richards, L.N. and Bengtson, V.L. (1991). Intergenerational solidarity in families. In S.P. Pfeifer and M.B. Sussman (Eds), *Families: Intergenerational and Generational Connections* (pp. 11–46). New York: Haworth Press.

Robinson, T., Callister, M., Magoffin, D. and Moore, J. (2007). The portrayal of older characters in Disney animated films. *Journal of Aging Studies*, 21(3), 203–13.

Rogers, C.R. (1959). A theory of therapy, personality and interpersonal relationships, as developed in the client-centered framework. In S. Koch (Ed.), *Psychology: A Study of Science* Vol. 3 (pp. 210–11; 184–256). New York: McGraw Hill.

Roman, A. (2006). *Deviating From the Standard: Effects on Labor Continuity and Career Patterns*. Amsterdam: Dutch University Press.

Roos, J.P. (2005). *Life's Turning Points and Generational Consciousness. Monograph*. Helsinki: University of Helsinki.

Rosenthal, C.J., Martin-Matthews, A. and Matthews, S.H. (1996). Caught in the middle? Occupancy in multiple roles and help to parents in national probability sample of Canadian adults. *The Journal of Gerontology*, 51B(6), S274–S83.

Rossi, A, and Rossi, P. (1990). *Of Human Bonding*. New York, NY: Aldine de Gruyter.

Rowe, J.W. and Kahn, R.L. (1987). Human aging: usual and successful. *Science*, 237(4811), 143–49.

Rowe, J.W. and Kahn, R.L. (1997). Successful aging. *The Gerontologist*, 37(4), 433–40.

Rowe, J.W. and Kahn, R.L. (1998). *Successful Aging*. New York: Pantheon.

Rubin, R.M. and White-Means, S.I. (2009). Informal caregiving: Dilemmas of sandwiched caregivers. *Journal of Family and Economic Issues*, 30(3), 252–67.

Ruth, J.E. and Coleman, P. (1996). Personality and aging. In J.E. Birren and K.W. Schaie (Eds), *Handbook of the Psychology of Aging*. London: Academic Press.

Sadler, E. and Biggs, S. (2006) Exploring the link between spirituality and successful ageing. *Journal of Social Work Practice*. 20(3), 267–80.

Salin, D. (2003). Ways of explaining workplace bullying: A review of enabling, motivating and precipitating structures and processes in the work environment. *Human Relations*, 56(10), 1213–32.

Samuels, A., Shorter, B. and Plaut, F. (1986). *A Critical Dictionary of Jungian Analysis.* London: Routledge and Kegan-Paul.

Sanchez, M. (2007). Spain's intergenerational awakening: New initiatives to promote intergenerational solidarity. *Journal of Intergenerational Relationships*, 5(2), 113–18.

Sanchez, M., Butts, D.M., Hatton-Yeo, A., Henkin, N.A., Jarrott, S.E., Kaplan, M.S., Martínez, A., Newman, S., Pinazo, S., Sáez, J., Weintraub, A.P.C. and Rodrígu, M.A. (2007). *Intergenerational Programmes.* Barcelona: la Caixa Foundation: Social Studies Collection No. 23.

Schaie, K.W. and Willis, S. (2002). *Aging and Old Age*. New York: Springer.

Schiamberg, L.B. and Gans, D. (2000). Elder abuse by adult children: An applied ecological framework for understanding contextual risk factors and the intergenerational character of quality of life. *International Journal of Aging and Human Development*, 50(4), 329–59.

Schneider, J.W. (1985). Social problems theory: The constructionist view. *Annual Review of Sociology*, 11, 209–29.

Schultz, H.J. (1999). Productive aging: An economist's view. In N. Morrow-Howell, J. Hinterlong and M. Sherraden (Eds), *Productive Aging: Concepts and Challenge*. Baltimore: The Johns Hopkins University Press.

Schulz, R. and Martire, L.M. (2004). Family caregiving of persons with dementia prevalence, health effects, and support strategies. *American Journal of Geriatric Psychiatry*, 12(3), 240–49.

Schwartz, L.K. and Simmons, J.P. (2001). Contact quality and attitudes toward the elderly. *Educational Gerontology*, 27, 127–37.

Schwartz, W. (2002). From passivity to competence: A conceptualization of knowledge, skill, tolerance, and empathy. *Psychiatry*, 65(4), 338–45.

Settersten, R. (2006). Linking the two ends of life: What Gerontology can learn from childhood studies. *Journal of Gerontology: Social Sciences*, B60(4), S173–S80.

Shaw, B.A., Krause, N., Liang, J. and Bennet, J. (2007). Tracking changes in social relations throughout late life. *The Journals of Gerontology Series B: Psychological Sciences and Social Sciences*, 62(2), S90–S9.

Shweder, R. (1998). *Welcome to Middle Age*. Chicago: UCP.

Sicker, M. (1994). The paradox of productive aging. *Aging International*, 21(2), 12–14.

Sidorenko, A. (2007). World policies on aging and the United Nations. In M. Robinson, W. Novelli, C. Pearson and L. Norris (Eds), *Global Health and Global Aging*. San Francisco: Jossey-Bass, pp. 3–14.

Sidorenko, A. and Walker, A. (2004). The Madrid International Plan of Action on Ageing: From conception to implementation. *Ageing and Society*, 24(2), 147–65.

Silverstein, M. and Bengtson, V.L. (1997). Intergenerational solidarity and the structure of adult-parent relationships. *American Journal of Sociology*, 103(2), 429–60.

Silverstein, M. and Litwak, E. (1993). A task specific typology of intergenerational family structure in later life. *The Gerontologist*, 33(2), 258–64.

Silverstein, M. and Marenco, A. (2001). How Americans enact the grandparent role? *Journal of Marriage and Family*, 22(4), 493–522.

Silverstein, M. and Parrott, T.M. (1997). Attitudes toward public support of the elderly. *Research on Aging*, 13(1), 108–32.

Silverstein, M., Gans, D. and Yang, F.M. (2006). Intergenerational support to aging parents: The role of norms and needs. *Journal of Family Issues*, 27(8), 1068–84.

Silverstein, M., Gans, D., Lowenstein, A., Giarrusso, R. and Bengtson, V.L. (2010). Older parent-child relationships in six nations: The intersection of affection and conflict. *Journal of Marriage and Family*, 72, 1006–21.

Skilton-Sylvester, E. and Garcia, A. (1998–1999). The intergenerational programs to address the challenge of immigration. *Generations*, 22(4), 58–63.

Small, N. (2007). Living well until you die. *Annals of the New York Academy of Sciences*, 1114, 194–203.

Smart, C. (2000). Stories of family life: Cohabitation, marriage and social change. *Canadian Journal of Family Law*, 20(1), 20–53.

Spiess, K. and Schneider, U. (2002). Midlife caregiving and employment: An analysis of adjustments in work hours and informal care for female employees in Europe (Economics Working Paper 009). *European Network of Economic Policy Research Institutes.*

SPReW project (2008). *Generational Approach to the Social Patterns of Relation to Work*, Executive summary, September.

Stacey, J. (1990). *Brave New Families: Stories of Domestic Upheaval in Late Twentieth Century America.* New York: Basic Books.

Stenner, P. and Taylor, D. (2008). Psychosocial welfare: Reflections on an emerging field. *Critical Social Policy*, 28(4), 415–37.

Stoller, E.P. and Miklowski, C.S. (2008). Spouses caring for spouses: Untangling the influence of relationship and gender. In M.E. Szinovacz and A. Davey (Eds), *Caregiving Contexts: Cultural, Familial and Societal Implications* (pp. 115–32). New York: Springer.

Stones, M.J. and Pittman, D. (1995). Individual differences in attitudes about elder abuse: The elder abuse attitudes test. *Canadian Journal on Aging*, 14(2), 61–71.

Strawbridge, W.J., Wallhagen, M.I. and Cohen, R.D. (2002). Successful aging and well being. *The Gerontologist*, 42(6), 727–33.

Stuifbergen, M., Van Delden, J. and Dykstra, P. (2008). The implications of today's family structures for support giving to older parents. *Ageing and Society*, 28(3), 413–34.

Sugarman, L. (2000). *Lifespan Development*. London: Taylor & Francis.

Szinovacz, M.E. (2007). Commentary: The future of intergenerational relationships – variability and vulnerabilities. In K.W. Schaie and P. Uhlenberg (Eds), *Social Structures: The Impact of Demographic Changes on the Well-Being of Older Persons* (pp. 262–82). New York: Springer.

Szinovacz, M.E. (2008). Children in caregiving families. In M.E. Szinovacz and A. Davey (Eds), *Caregiving Contexts: Cultural, Familial and Societal Implications* (pp. 161–94). New York: Springer.

Tate, R.B., Lah, L. and Cuddy, T.E. (2003). Definition of successful aging by elderly Canadian males: The Manitoba follow-up study. *The Gerontologist*, 43, 735–44.

Taylor, A.S., LoSciuto, L., Fox, M., Hilbert, S.M. and Sonkowsky, M. (1999). The mentoring factor: Evaluation of the Across Ages' intergenerational approach to drug abuse prevention. *Child and Youth Services*, 20(1–2), 77–99.

Taylor, C. (1989). *Sources of the Self.* Cambridge, MA: Harvard University.

Thomas, E., McGarty, C. and Mavor, K. (2009). Aligning identities, emotions and beliefs to create commitment to sustainable social and political action. *Personality and Social Psychology Review*, 13(3), 194–218.

Tinker, A., Manthorpe, J. and Biggs, S. (2010). Elder mistreatment and neglect. In H.M. Fillit, K. Rockwood and K. Woodhouse (Eds), *Brocklehurst's Textbook of Geriatric Medicine and Gerontology* (pp. 307–12). Kidlington: Saunders.

Tomassini, C., Glaser, K., Wolf, D., Broese van Grenou, M. and Grundy, E. (2004). Living arrangements among older people: An overview of trends in Europe and the USA. *Population Trends*, 115, 24–34.

Tornstam, L. (1996). Gerotranscendence: A theory about maturing into old age. *Journal of Aging and Identity*, 1(1), 37–50.

Tornstam, L. (2003). *Gerotranscendence From Young Old to Old Old Age.* Online publication from the Social Gerontology Group, Uppsala.

Tornstam, L. (2005). *Gerotranscendence.* New York: Springer.

Turner, B.S. (1998). Ageing and generational conflicts. *British Journal of Sociology*, 49(2), 299–304.

Turner, B.S. (2002). The distaste of taste: Bourdieu, cultural capital and the Australian postwar elite. *Journal of Consumer Culture*, 2(2), 219–40.

United Nations (1982). *Report of the First World Assembly on Ageing: Vienna International Plan of Action* (p. 24).

United Nations (1983). *Vienna International Plan of Action on Ageing.* New York: United Nations.

United Nations (1995). *Report of the World Summit on Social Development.* A/CONF.166/9. April 16. New York: United Nations.

United Nations (2002). *Report of the Second World Assembly on Ageing: Madrid Political Declaration and International Plan of Action* 2002 (p. 79).

United Nations (2003). *UN Youth Report.* New York: United Nations.

Vaillant, G.E. (1990). Avoiding negative life outcomes: Evidence from a forty five year study. In P.B. Baltes and M.M. Baltes (Eds), *Successful Aging. Perspectives from the Social Sciences.* New York: Cambridge University Press.

Vaillant, G.E. (2002). *Aging Well.* Boston: Little, Brown and Co.

Van den Hoonaard, D. (2009). Widowers' strategies of self-representation during research interviews: A sociological analysis. *Ageing and Society*, 29(2), 257–76.

Van Der Ven, K. (1999). Intergenerational theory: The missing element in today's intergenerational programs. In V. S. Kuehne (Ed.), *Understanding What We Have Created* (pp. 33–47). Binghamton: The Haworth Press.

Van Gaalen, R.I. and Dykstra, P.A. (2006). Solidarity and conflict between adult children and parents: A latent class analysis. *Journal of Marriage and Family*, 68(4), 947–60.

Vendramin, P. (2004). Le travail au singulier – Le lien social à l'épreuve de l'*individualisation*, Louvain-la-Neuve: Académia Bruylant: Paris L'Harmattan.

Vendramin P. (Ed.) (2008). Changing social patterns of relation to work – Qualitative approach through biographies and group interviews, Report of the SPReW projet (CIT5–028048), 6PC, European Commission, DG Research, 2008a. Downloadable: http://www.ftunamur.org/sprew.

Vendramin, P. (2009). *Age Diversity and Intergenerational Relationships at the Workplace.* Paper presented at the 4th conference Young People and Societies in Europe and around the Mediterranean, Forlì, March 2009.

Ventura-Merkel, C. and Liddoff, L. (1983). *Program Innovation in Aging: Community Planning for Intergenerational Programming*. Washington, DC: National Council on Aging. 8.

Villar, F. (2007). Intergenerational or multigenerational? A question of nuance. *Journal of Intergenerational Relationships*, 5(1): 115–17.

Vincent, J.A. (2005). Understanding generations: Political economy and culture in an ageing society. *The British Journal of Sociology*, 56(4), 579–99.

Visker, R. (1995). *Michel Foucault: Genealogy as Critique*. London: Verso.

Voydanoff, P. (2005). Social integration, work-family conflict and facilitation and job and marital quality. *Journal of Marriage and Family*, 67(3), 666–79.

Wade-Benzoni, K.A. (2008). Maple trees and weeping willows: The role of time, uncertainty, and affinity in intergenerational decisions. *Negotiation and Conflict Management Research*, 1, 220–45.

Wade-Benzoni, K. and Tost, L. (2009). The egoism and altruism of intergenerational behaviour. *Personality and Social Psychology Review*, 13(2), 165–93.

Wakabayashi, C. and Donato, K.M. (2006). Does caregiving increase poverty among women in later life? Evidence from the health and retirement survey. *Journal of Health and Social Behavior*, 47(3), 258–74.

Walker, A. (2006) Active ageing in employment: Its meaning and potential. *Asia-Pacific Review*, 13(1), 78–93.

Walker, A.J. (Ed.) (1996). *The New Generational Contract*. London: UCL Press.

Walker, A.J. (2000a). Sharing long-term care between the family and the state – a European perspective. In W.T. Liu and H. Kendig (Eds), *Who Should Care for the Elderly?* (pp. 78–106). Singapore: Singapore University Press.

Walker, A.J. (2000b). Aging in Europe. *Hallym International Journal of Aging*, 2(1), 27–39.

Walker, A.J. and Lowenstein, A. (2009). European perspective on quality of life in old age. *European Journal of Aging*, 6(2), 61–66.

Walker, A.J., Pratt, C.C. and Eddy, L. (1995). Informal caregiving to aging family members. *Family Relations*, 44(4), 402–11.

Ward, R.A. (2008). Multiple parent-adult child relations and well-being in middle and later life. *Journal of Gerontology: Social Sciences*, 63B(4), S239–S47.

Weaver, R. (1973). *The Wise Old Woman*. New York: Shambhala.

Weigert, A.J. (1991). *Mixed Emotions*. New York: State University Press.

Weigert, A.J. and Hastings, R. (1977). Identity loss, family, and social change. *American Journal of Sociology*, 82(6), 1171–85.

Westerhof, G. and Barrett, A. (2005). Age identity and subjective well-being. *Journal of Gerontology: Social Sciences*, 60B(3), S129–36.

Wikipedia. http://en.wikipedia.org/wiki/Empathy (23/6/09: 1).

Wilkinson, R. and Pickett, K. (2009). *The Spirit Level: Why More Equal Societies Almost Always Do Better.* London: Allen Lane.

Willetts, D. (2010). *The Pinch: How the Baby-Boomers Took Their Children's Future*. London: Atlantic Books.

Williams, A. and Nussbaum, J.F. (2001). *Intergenerational Communication Across the Life Span*. Mahwah. NJ: Lawrence Erlbaum Associates.

Williams, B., Sawyer, S. and Wahlstrom, C. (2005). *Marriages, Families and Intimate Relationships*. Boston, MA: Pearson.

Williamson, J.B., Watts-Roy, D.M. and Kingson, E.R. (1999). *The Generational Equity Debate*. New York: Columbia University Press.

Willson, A.E., Shuey K.M. and Elder G.H .Jr (2003). Ambivalence in the relationship of adult children to aging parents and in-laws. *Journal of Marriage and Family*, 65(4), 1055–72.

Willson, A., Shuey, K.M., Elder, G.H. Jr. and Wickrama, K.A.S. (2006). Ambivalence in mother-adult child relations: A dyadic analysis. *Social Psychology Quarterly*, 69(3), 235–52.

Wisensale, S. (2008). Caregiving policy in the United States: Addressing the needs of caregivers of the elderly. In R. Hudson (Ed.), *Boomer Bust?* Lexington, MA: Greenwood Press.

Wolff, J.L. and Kasper, J.D. (2006). Caregivers of frail elders: Updating a national profile. *The Gerontologist*, 46(3), 344–56.

Woodward, K. (1991). *Aging and its Discontents: Freud and Other Fictions*. Indianapolis, IN: Indiana University Press.

Woodward, K. (1995). Tribute to the older woman. In M. Featherstone and A. Wernick (Eds), *Images of Ageing*. London: Routledge.

Woodward, K. (1999). *Figuring Age: Women, Bodies, Generations*. Bloomington and Indianapolis, IN: Indiana University Press.

Woolfe, R. and Biggs, S. (1998). Counselling older adults: Issues and awareness. *Psychology Quarterly*, 10(2), 189–94.

World Health Organization (2002a). *Active Ageing: A Policy Framework*. Second World Assembly on Aging. Madrid: Spain.

World Health Organization (2002b). *Missing Voices: Views of Older Persons on Elder Abuse*. Geneva: WHO.

World Health Organization (2007). *World Health Statistics 2007*. Geneva: WHO.

World Health Organization (2008). *Age-Friendly Cities*. Geneva: WHO.

Zeldin, S., McDaniel, A.K., Topitzest, D. and Calvert, M. (2000). *Youth in Decision-Making: A Study on the Impacts of Youth on Adults and Organizations*. Chevy Chase, MD: Innovation Center for Community and Youth Development, National 4-h Council.

Zemke, R., Raines C. and Filipczack, B. (2000). *Generations at Work: Managing the Clash of Veterans, Boomers, Xers and Nexters in your Workplace*. New York: AMACOM.

Index

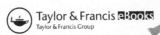